The Truth about Telehealth

The Truth about Telehealth

Why a Revolutionary Industry Has Failed to Deliver and How It Can Still Be a Game-Changer for Healthcare

Larry D. Jones

© 2018 Larry D. Jones

All rights reserved. No part of this publication may be reproduced, distributed, or transmitted in any form or by any means, including photocopying, recording, or other electronic or mechanical methods, without the prior written permission of the publisher, except in the case of brief quotations embodied in critical reviews and certain other noncommercial uses permitted by copyright law.

ISBN-13: 9781981890361
ISBN-10: 198189036X
Library of Congress Control Number: 2018900358
CreateSpace Independent Publishing Platform
North Charleston, South Carolina

Table of Contents

Introduction xiii

Chapter 1   Our Current System Is Broken 1

    Rising Costs 2

    Growing Inconvenience 4

    Increasing Dissatisfaction 6

    It's Time for Change 8

Chapter 2   What Is Telehealth 11

    Synchronous 12

    Asynchronous 13

        Remote Patient Monitoring ⋯⋯⋯⋯⋯⋯ 15

        Telehealth Applications Working Together ⋯⋯ 17

        Recent Developments in Telehealth ⋯⋯⋯⋯ 17

Chapter 3 **Telemedicine versus Telehealth** ⋯⋯⋯⋯⋯ **21**

        History of the Words "Telemedicine" and

        "Telehealth" ⋯⋯⋯⋯⋯⋯⋯⋯⋯⋯⋯⋯ 22

        Formal Definitions ⋯⋯⋯⋯⋯⋯⋯⋯⋯⋯ 25

        Other Terms ⋯⋯⋯⋯⋯⋯⋯⋯⋯⋯⋯⋯ 27

        Our Conclusions ⋯⋯⋯⋯⋯⋯⋯⋯⋯⋯⋯ 28

Chapter 4 **The Promise of Telehealth** ⋯⋯⋯⋯⋯⋯ **31**

        Helps Individuals ⋯⋯⋯⋯⋯⋯⋯⋯⋯⋯ 32

        A Solution for Employers ⋯⋯⋯⋯⋯⋯⋯ 35

        The Reality of Telehealth Today ⋯⋯⋯⋯⋯ 37

Chapter 5 **Why Aren't Brokers Selling Telehealth?** ⋯⋯ **39**

        Benefits Brokers: The Basics ⋯⋯⋯⋯⋯⋯ 39

              "Not Worth My Time" 42

              Workplace Wellness 45

              Demand More 45

Chapter 6 Finding a Solution that Works 49

              Is Your Solution Working? 50

              What Brokers *Should* Be Looking For 52

              Employers Beware 55

Chapter 7 Health Insurance Companies and

              Their Telehealth Solutions 57

              How Insurance Companies' Telehealth

              Solutions Operate 58

              They Don't Care If People Use It 60

              The Real Cost to Employers 62

              Employees Get Screwed 63

              You Get What You Pay For 65

Chapter 8 Why You Shouldn't Dump Telehealth on HR · · 67

    HR Is Sick of Employee Benefits· · · · · · · · · · · 68

    HR Is Not Marketing · · · · · · · · · · · · · · · · · · · 70

    Who Is Accountable for Results? · · · · · · · · · · · · 72

    Set Yourself Up for Success · · · · · · · · · · · · · · · 74

Chapter 9 Telehealth Needs Executive Engagement · · · · 75

    Executives Need to Be Involved in the

    Decision Making· 76

    Executives Need to Be Telehealth Champions · · 78

    Working Directly with Telehealth Providers · · · 80

    A Call to Action for CEOs and CFOs· · · · · · · · · 82

Chapter 10 Are All Telehealth Companies the Same? · · · · 83

    Fee per Use versus Zero Co-Pay · · · · · · · · · · · · 84

    Limited versus Unlimited Consultations · · · · · · 85

    Employee Only versus Entire Family· · · · · · · · · 86

Claims versus No Claims 87

No Accountability versus Accountability 88

Good versus Bad User Experience 89

It All Comes Down to Utilization 91

Chapter 11 Objections to Telehealth **93**

The Physician-Patient Relationship 93

Continuity of Care 95

Quality of Care 96

Information Security 98

There Are No Real Concerns 99

Chapter 12 Telehealth FAQs **101**

Who Are the Doctors? 101

When Should I Use Telehealth? 103

Is the Quality of Care as Good? 104

How Do I Access a Telehealth Doctor? 104

How Do Prescriptions Work? · · · · · · · · · · · · · 105

How Much Does Telehealth Cost? · · · · · · · · · · 106

What Limits Are There? · · · · · · · · · · · · · · · · · 107

Is Telehealth Private and Secure? · · · · · · · · · · · 108

Chapter 13 How to Choose Between an On-Site Clinic and Telehealth · · · · · · · · · · · · · · · · · · 109

Availability · 110

Available Services · 112

Implementation · 113

Savings and Value · 115

Telehealth Comes Out Ahead · · · · · · · · · · · · · 116

Chapter 14 How Telehealth Is Transforming Health Care · 117

Different Site of Care Needs · · · · · · · · · · · · · · 117

Increased Competition · · · · · · · · · · · · · · · · · 121

Changing Regulations · · · · · · · · · · · · · · · · · 123

Health Care of the Future · · · · · · · · · · · · · · · 125

Chapter 15 Telepsychiatry - An Industry in Need · · · · · · **127**

How Telepsychiatry Works · · · · · · · · · · · · · · 129

Telepsychiatry in Schools and Colleges · · · · · · 131

Telepsychiatry in Prisons · · · · · · · · · · · · · · · · 133

Telepsychiatry for the Mildly to Moderately Ill · · 134

Therapy on Demand · · · · · · · · · · · · · · · · · · · 136

Chapter 16 Other Emerging Specialties · · · · · · · · · · · · · **137**

Physical Therapy · 137

Dentistry · 140

Optometry · 142

Access to Specialties Improves Access to Care · · 145

Chapter 17 The Future of Telehealth · · · · · · · · · · · · · · · **147**

Integration versus New Providers · · · · · · · · · · 148

New Services · 150

Remote Data Collection · · · · · · · · · · · · · · · · · 151

The Possibilities of Big Data · · · · · · · · · · · · · · 153

Conclusion · 154

About the Author · 157

References · 159

Introduction

Technology has revolutionized almost every industry in the modern world. It changes the way we drive, the way we communicate, the way we eat and sleep, and even the fabric of the traditional eight-to-five workdays. It is hard to imagine not being able to instantly text or call someone on the other side of the country or not being able to check your e-mail while in the car. Almost every aspect of modern life has been made faster and more convenient through telecommunications technology - except health care.

Even as technology has improved, access to health care has worsened for many Americans. The Affordable Care Act may have increased the number of people with health insurance, but the fact is that health care remains unaffordable and inconvenient for most people. An increasing percentage of health insurance plans have expensive premiums, sky-high deductibles, and costly co-pays. People are paying for care that they can hardly afford to use. Plus, physician shortages mean absurdly long wait times, especially in crowded cities. Patients are resorting to urgent cares and emergency rooms, making care even more expensive. Patients in rural areas face an even greater challenge: rural hospitals are closing, meaning long drive times and limited access to specialists in their area. Employers are also struggling with rising costs. Unable to sustain their current benefit levels, they have been forced to reduce benefits and shift healthcare costs to employees through higher premiums, deductibles, and co-pays. Technological advances have done little to help these worrying trends. But there is a solution that could help millions of Americans get more affordable, convenient access to care: telehealth.

"Telehealth," put simply, means using telecommunications technology to provide remote care. The term encompasses any use of telecommunications technology in the medical field, even faxing a prescription to a pharmacy, but typically when people use the word "telehealth" or "telemedicine," they are talking about virtual doctor visits. With these telehealth services, patients can call or videoconference with a doctor instead of going into a physicians' office, urgent care, or other site of care. The doctors can diagnose, treat, and manage illnesses and other medical conditions remotely. This lowers the overall cost to deliver care as well as reduces the total time involved for the patient and provider. Telehealth brings the medical care *to* the patient, wherever they are. It enables patients to get the care they need, without sacrificing valuable time or money to get it.

Back in the late 2000s, I saw the potential that telehealth had to transform the landscape of health care. It could be a disrupter on the same magnitude as Uber for public transportation. But no one had yet created a solution that actually worked for the patients who needed it most. I even sat down with another big telehealth company and discussed their solution with them. Coming from a health care and software engineering background, I had ideas for what could be changed to improve the user experience, but there was no interest at the moment. However, I knew there was an opportunity, and in 2009, TelaCare Health Solutions was born. My mission was to provide convenient, cost-effective, high-quality care through virtual health consultations. I created a solution that works, providing a solid ROI for employers *and* a valuable benefit to employees.

In the years since TelaCare Health Solutions started, the company and the industry have continued to grow. But the industry has not yet fulfilled its promise of transforming health care. While more people have access to a telehealth solution than ever before, use of the solutions has not taken off like predicted. In fact, utilization of telehealth solutions is shockingly low. Having been in the industry, I have seen firsthand the challenges that telehealth still needs to overcome for it to become an integral part of our health care system. And the number-one problem that telehealth is facing is *education*.

Being out at conferences, brokers' offices, and employers, I have realized how few people actually understand telehealth. Many have heard the term, but no one really knows what it is, how to use it, when to use it, or why you would even want to use it. As a passionate supporter of telehealth, it can be frustrating to see this lack of awareness. Telehealth has a multitude of benefits for employers and individuals, especially considering its low cost. How many HR solutions are there that can directly lower an employer's health care costs *and* employees' individual health care spending? All while reducing sick time

→ *Telehealth as a solution*

and paid time off (PTO) due to doctors' visits? Telehealth solutions can solve some of the most pressing problems that individuals and employers face in the current system, namely, rising costs and increased time spent getting care. Telehealth is a remarkable solution that has the potential to reduce the total cost of care, improve access and equity of access to care across the country, and improve overall quality of care and health outcomes. But still, brokers often fail to mention the solution, employers do not ask for it, and individuals never hear about it. Many people do not even know what they are missing.

The problem is especially acute at small to midsized employers. Unfortunately, due to their size, many of the larger telehealth companies do not care to win their business. They are not knocking on these employers' doors to tell them about telehealth. And these companies also often use smaller local brokers that do not have the breadth of resources and internal education that the largest brokers have. But telehealth is a solution that works for companies of all sizes. There is no fixed cost that makes it too expensive for small employers to justify. It is a simple flat per-employee-per-month fee. At TelaCare, we even have a direct-to-consumer solution because it makes just as much sense for an individual to buy it as for a company. There is no reason that small or midsized companies and their employees should be left out of telehealth.

The second biggest problem that telehealth is facing is *bad solutions*. There are actually many employers that already provide telehealth solutions to their employees. In the 2016 Willis Towers Watson Employee Benefits survey, 70 percent of large employers offered telehealth. But utilization across all of these companies is around 3 percent.[1] That is dismal. There is no other way to put it. But the problem is not with the concept. The problem is that the majority of the solutions currently in the market are ineffective. The biggest players have not innovated or developed a solution that works. Instead, they have relied on venture capital investment to sustain their businesses. Unfortunately, these companies have managed to stay at the top of the industry because most brokers and employers are treating telehealth as a commodity. After all, the basic premise of the solution is simple: the patient picks up the phone, calls the telehealth number, and is connected to a US board-certified doctor. The patient describes the symptoms, and then the doctor diagnoses and recommends treatment. How many variations could there be?

This attitude does telehealth a disservice and is a leading contributor to the low utilization many of these solutions have. In fact, there are many small but key differences in telehealth solutions that determine its success. Do you want a solution that merely "checks the box" but is never used and never saves anyone any money? Or do you want a solution that directly lowers employers' health care costs, increases employee productivity, and provides a meaningful benefit for employees? At TelaCare Health Solutions, I have figured out how to remove the barriers to utilization *and* how to educate people on the solution. That is why my solution averages over 30 percent utilization for our clients. There is a huge gap between outcomes from different telehealth providers, and more people need to know about how to get results from telehealth.

The goal of this book is to help educate individuals and employers on telehealth and how to choose the right solution. The fact is that *most* of the solutions on the market are ineffective, because health insurers, big telehealth companies, and brokers can get away with providing a bad solution. Right now, most employers and individuals do not know what questions to ask or what to look for. They have to rely on outside groups, mostly brokers, to provide the best advice. And clearly where telehealth is concerned, these resources are falling short. That is why I am here to pull back the curtain on telehealth. There is a solution out there that can help you. It is not expensive, and it is not hard to implement. Savings can start as soon as you sign up. But not just any telehealth provider will do. You need to know how to evaluate telehealth providers and why you cannot rely on your broker or your health insurer to provide the best solution. Telehealth can change health care for the better. But we need good solutions that drive utilization if we want to see results.

CHAPTER 1

Our Current System Is Broken

It's no surprise that our current health care system isn't working for everyone. And the list of problems is long. Getting quality medical care is expensive, time consuming, confusing, and stressful. Even a visit to your primary care doctor isn't always easy anymore. But quality medical care is important. It improves our health, our wallets, and our happiness. Illness and injury is already stressful enough; health care shouldn't add to the burden.

The government has been involved in health care for decades, but the increasing challenges of providing quality affordable care have prompted the government to intervene even more. This led to the passing of the Affordable Care Act and mandating electronic health records. Whether you agree with these measures or not, no one can disagree that there are still challenges with these new legislations. Health care costs continue to rise, access is more inconvenient, and people are becoming more dissatisfied with their medical care.

Rising Costs

Premiums and fees have risen dramatically in recent years for those who don't qualify for government subsidies. On the public exchange for 2017, the average individual premium was $393 per month and the average family premium was $1,021 per month. And premiums are expected to continue to rise in coming years. That's not what most people would call "affordable." The premiums aren't the only cost barrier on the public exchange. Too often, families are paying more for less coverage. These already-expensive plans usually have higher deductibles than plans of the past, leaving the insured to cover the costs for almost all of their medical care. Doctors and hospitals often demand that you pay up front before receiving care. The estimate might even be higher than what you actually need to pay, but there's no way to know until you actually receive the bill. In reality, these plans aren't much more than expensive catastrophic plans that will benefit only those who have devastating accidents or illnesses.

For those who are lucky enough to have employer-provided health care coverage, the increases have been more modest but still very real. Employers simply cannot carry all of the cost of increased premiums. They are passing these costs on to their employees through higher premiums and increased co-pays and deductibles. An annual study by the Kaiser Family Foundation found that 67 percent of employees face a co-payment when they visit a primary care. Additionally, the number of employees facing a deductible of greater than $1,000 for single-person coverage has grown from 22 percent in 2009 to 51 percent in 2016.[2]

Employers are also using different plan options to shift some of the burden of rising medical costs on to their employees. In recent years, more and more employers are offering High Deductible Health Plans, or HDHPs, in an effort to shift more of the costs to employees. HDHPs, when used correctly, can be beneficial, especially to the young and healthy. But compared to the PPO (Preferred Provider Organizations) plans more popular in the past, they are like the 401(k) compared to the pension plan. HDHPs have lower monthly premiums, which is enticing to employees. But the deductibles are high, and many employees find themselves unable to pay when an expensive medical bill comes in the mail. PPOs, on the other hand, have slightly higher monthly premiums and lower deductibles. People tend to want more money in their pocket *now* but are then unprepared for future costs. Employers, recognizing this, are pushing the HDHPs to save themselves money and instead make their employees responsible for their own care.

The truth is that yes, the Affordable Care Act covered millions that previously couldn't afford health insurance. But everyone else has to cover those costs, and it's putting health insurance financially out of reach for people who previously *could* pay. Insurance is now more expensive and less comprehensive than before. People are finding themselves on the line for expensive co-pays or up-front payment when seeking medical care. For many middle-class Americans, the current system is simply unaffordable.

Growing Inconvenience

In addition to rising costs, health care is becoming more inconvenient. Wait times to see a doctor can be weeks, appointments take too long, and too often people have to resort to urgent cares and emergency rooms for nonurgent care. People's time is too valuable to waste getting medical care. But there aren't really many other options.

There is a physician shortage in the United States, and the gap between supply and demand is getting worse. The demand for medical care is increasing faster than recruitment of new doctors can keep up. The 2017 Association of American Medical Colleges Physician Supply and Demand report showed that by 2030, there will be a shortfall of 7,300 to 43,100 primary care physicians.[3] There are many factors, including an aging population, dissatisfaction with the ACA and EHR (electronic health records), and burdensome education, insurance, and certification requirements. As our population grows older, many older doctors are retiring, and the increasing requirements to become a doctor means that there aren't enough young doctors to fill their positions. Not to mention that the elderly require more medical care. All of this simply means that for the average consumer, it's *hard to get an appointment.*

Current wait times to see a primary care physician is about nineteen days. That's fine for your annual check-up, but it's not very helpful when you're sick. Plus, some insurance companies require that you see a primary care physician before you see a specialist. That means that even if you know you need to see an ENT doctor (ears-nose-throat), you'll have to wait first a couple of weeks to see your primary care. Then they'll refer you to the specialist, which could take another couple of weeks. With wait times this long, people are turning to urgent care and emergency rooms to get the care they need. Unfortunately, these are not the best sites of care for nonemergency medical conditions.

First, they are significantly more expensive. A visit to the urgent care is likely double what you'd pay at the physician office. And the emergency room can be as much as five times as expensive. Second, while you can visit these centers on the same day you have symptoms, the wait times can still be long and unpredictable. There are no designated appointment times, and they don't operate on a first-come, first-serve basis. Cases that are more urgent than yours will be seen first, so you may be in for a long day. And third, visiting these centers for nonurgent needs takes time and resources away from the staff providing emergency care to those who truly need it. But with limited other options, these are still popular centers of choice for people who need care *now*, not in a few weeks.

Even when you get an appointment, the process isn't fast and easy. The average doctor's visit takes three to four hours from start to finish. And most of that time is spent driving to the appointment, checking in, filling out paperwork, meeting with the nurse, and, of course, waiting. It's not spent with the actual physician. In fact, the 2016 Medscape Physician Compensation Report found that 56 percent of male and 49 percent of female physicians spend less than seventeen minutes with each patient.[4]

People are spending a major chunk of their day to spend a minuscule amount of time with their actual doctor.

These inconveniences in accessing care really add up. People don't have the time to spend hours going to the doctor. And the more people in your family, the more these inconveniences multiply. Caring for others is a fact of life, whether it's an elderly parent, a spouse, or children. Every time someone has to take time off work to take themselves or a loved one to the doctor, they have to use PTO or work extra another day.

Increasing Dissatisfaction

As if the rising costs and growing inconvenience of medical care weren't enough, people are becoming increasingly dissatisfied with the care that they do receive. The system seems stacked against them, and physicians are less relational than in the past.

Contributing to the dissatisfaction is the confusion around medical billing and the lack of transparency. If you've ever received a surprise medical bill or a bill you didn't understand, you're not alone. A Consumer Reports study in 2015 found that one in three privately insured Americans have had a surprise medical bill.[5] Medical billing is complicated, so there are many ways that these surprise bills can happen.

You may know to look for an in-network hospital. But just because the hospital is in-network doesn't mean your physician is. Insurance companies contract with hospitals, but the hospital may contract *independently* with a physician that accepts different insurance. While uncommon in an evaluative appointment, it can easily happen during a surgery or in the emergency room. If you go in for surgery with one in-network doctor, but he needs to call in another surgeon for help or a second opinion, that second physician may be out of network. You might never even know—until you get your bill, that is. You'll get hit with a big out-of-network charge for that surgeon's help, without any of your approval or even knowledge.

Medical errors are also more common than you might think. In fact, an audit of insurance companies found that over 90 percent of medical bills contained errors. These errors can be everything from accidentally double billing a procedure, incorrectly counting quantities of medications, and the wrong amount of time recorded under anesthesia, to name a few. And it's almost impossible for the average consumer to find and identify these errors. Most medical bills don't contain an itemized report of charges; you have to request them. Even then, medical bills are filled with codes for different procedures, which vary by insurance company. Unless you or a friend is a certified medical bill coder, you may be out of luck. Even when you spot an error, you then have to get the hospital to agree to change it and resubmit the claim to your insurance company. Because of the difficulty involved in finding and correcting billing errors, most consumers end up just paying the bill, even if they disagree with it.

Patients are also becoming more dissatisfied with the patient experience. Long wait times at the doctor's office lead to frazzled and annoyed patients, who often just want to leave the doctor's office as quickly as possible. And the doctors are trying to move on to the next patient quickly, too. So instead of open dialogue with lots of questions and answers, communication is harried and brief. Patients may skip questions they meant to ask when facing a doctor who is trying to get out the door. Or they may forget the doctor's instructions as soon as they're said. Adding to the trouble is the mountain of documentation that is required of doctors as part of electronic health records (EHRs) and other programs. EHRs in particular have had many positive impacts on health care but have unintentionally created a divide during appointments. Physicians often bring computers into the room, so they can enter the required data during the visit, but physicians are now spending more time on the computer than actually interacting with patients. In an already-short visit, one study found that doctors with EHRs in the exam room spend 33 percent of their time looking at the computer instead of the patient. And the problem is likely only going to get worse. A study on doctors in training, or residents, found that residents spend only an average of eight minutes per patient per day, with over half of their time spent in front of a computer. There's nothing more frustrating than spending hours to see a doctor, only to feel like you didn't even have a chance to really communicate.

It's Time for Change

The medical industry is slow to change, so the problems continue to get worse. And consumers are getting upset. People simply cannot afford the time or money that traditional health care requires.

Luckily, innovation in medical care is happening. New technologies, new treatment options, and consumer demands are all helping reform medical care. While no single solution will solve every problem, meaningful change can happen. Telemedicine is one of these technologies.

CHAPTER 2

What Is Telehealth

The basic concept of telehealth is simple: health care professionals and organizations using telecommunications technology to deliver services to patients remotely. While it may seem like a new, hot topic in health care, in reality telehealth has been around in some form since the early 1900s. That is because the term "telehealth" covers all remote health care communication using telecommunications technology. As soon as the telephone and telegraph were invented, they have been used to send messages about medical care from a doctor or physician to a patient. But as new and improved telecommunications technologies developed, so have the applications and functionality of telehealth. This broad term now encompasses many different services and technologies. But while we're a long way from the first telephone and telegraph messages, many of the core functionalities of telehealth have remained. It is still used to provide more convenient service to remote patients. To categorize the many different types of telehealth, three broad groupings based on the core functions have been established: synchronous, store-and-forward/asynchronous, and remote patient monitoring

(RPM). We will discuss all three categories as well as recent telehealth technologies and how they fit into this structure.

Synchronous

Synchronous telehealth simply means that the provider, that is, the doctor or nurse, and the patient are communicating *at the same time,* even though they are not in the same location. Examples are a telephone call or videoconference. Synchronous telehealth is what most people are thinking of when they hear the words "telehealth" or "telemedicine." It is direct communication and conversation with a health care professional, similar to what would occur during a regular in-person visit.

The earliest form of consumer-based telehealth, the telephone, would be synchronous. The telephone was the start of the modern, connected world. Anyone with a telephone could connect to anyone, anywhere there was another telephone installed. This meant that patients and doctors could now easily reach each other, and doctors and specialists could communicate and share information as well. It allowed doctors to check in on how a patient's recommended treatment was going or for a concerned patient to ask any follow-up questions after a visit. It was especially useful in remote or rural areas where there may not have been a doctor nearby. Even though this was the earliest form of telehealth, it is still common today. Have you ever called your doctor's office for a prescription refill or to ask a question about medication instructions? How about calling your child's pediatrician the first time they have a fever? Or 911 in an emergency? These are all examples of telehealth innovations that have made accessing health care more convenient and efficient. But the telephone is so ubiquitous in today's society that we often forget that it is a telecommunications technology.

For synchronous telehealth interactions, there are two major technological developments that have improved communication: mobile phones and video calling. With mobile phones, patients can now be reached no matter where they are, greatly increasing the likelihood of the doctor reaching the patient on the first try. Before, the doctor may have had to schedule a call or try multiple times to reach someone. With video calling, a doctor or provider can actually see the patient and his or her condition, even though they're not in the same room. Instead of simply trying to describe a rash, for example, the doctor can see the markings and make more accurate diagnoses and treatment recommendations.

Asynchronous

Asynchronous telehealth is the opposite of synchronous—it is remote communication that happens at independent times for the health provider and the patient. Examples are e-mails, voicemails, and faxes. It is also called "store-and-forward," meaning that the information is stored somewhere, such as physical paper or e-mail, and then forwarded to someone else via telecommunications technology. The origins of telehealth are rooted in asynchronous communication. Doctors would send images data, images, and scans from one doctor or hospital to another to help with diagnoses and to help educate. The first major department within the hospital to embrace telehealth was the radiology department. The radiology department is in charge of x-rays, CT scans, MRIs, ultrasounds, and other imaging. These images would be sent to radiologists in other locations.

Due to the equipment and training needed, asynchronous telehealth occurred mainly in the hospital until the fax machine became widespread. Once the general public had fax machines, they could also use the store-and-forward method of telehealth to send or receive data from the hospital. But the next big invention for consumer store-and-forward telehealth was more impactful: voice mail. Voice mail became popular in the 1980s and allowed a telephone caller to leave a message if the recipient didn't pick up. It may be hard to remember a time without voice mail, but it actually wasn't that long ago. Before, the doctor had to reach you at a convenient time to discuss something over the phone. With voice mail, the doctor can give you the information whether you pick up or not. Voice mail is still widely used in health care communications today. If you think back to your last doctor's appointment, you probably had to provide a phone number and check a box to determine if the doctor could leave test results via voice mail. It adds even more convenience to the telephone by eliminating the need for the two people to be available at the same time.

However, the biggest development for store-and-forward telehealth has certainly been the advent of the Internet and e-mail. The major benefits of the Internet and e-mail are the ability to asynchronously send documents as well as the storage and search capabilities. Hospitals and doctors' offices now typically all have websites, many with patient portals that store patient-specific information. Patients can log in to their secure portal and download any documents they might need. It may also show a history of appointments and have a built-in scheduler to schedule future appointments. All of this information is uploaded by the provider to be accessed at a later time by patients, but it is stored indefinitely, and patients can access it as many times as they'd like. E-mail can also be used to communicate more directly with a patient. E-mail is often used to send test results or appointment reminders. Asynchronous communication, especially with the Internet and e-mail, has provided enormous benefits to both providers and patients by allowing both parties to communicate at a time that works best for them.

Remote Patient Monitoring

The last type of telehealth is also the newest: remote patient monitoring, or RPM. RPM uses advanced technology to gather patient health data outside of the traditional health care settings. This data is then transmitted wirelessly to a health care setting, where it is either analyzed by a computer program or an individual. The data is used to identify trends or specific incidents that can reduce hospitalizations and readmissions by providing more timely care. Some of the types of data collected are heart rate, weight, blood pressure, blood sugar, blood oxygen levels, and electrocardiograms.

An example of a common use of RPM is for monitoring falls in elderly people that live at home. Sensors can be attached to either the individual or their mobility devices, such as canes and walkers. The sensors can monitor location, gait, horizontal speed, and vertical acceleration to both predict the likelihood of a fall and to alert caregivers if the individual has fallen. This information can help keep the elderly at home longer, while still providing peace of mind that help will come if needed. RPM technology is also incorporated into many implantable pacemakers and defibrillators, so critical data can be continuously monitored. In fact, the CONNECT study (Clinical Evaluation of Remote Notification to Reduce Time to Clinical Decision) showed that implantable cardiac devices that actively transmitted data enabled physicians to make treatment decisions 17.4 days sooner than those who relied on reviewing the data during in-office visits. RPM technologies such as these enable physicians and individuals to be better informed about overall health, to ask better questions, and to make better recommendations and treatment plans.

While traditional RPM is sent automatically to a remote medical setting for analysis and assessment, a new type of RPM is emerging with personal electronic devices. Using smartphone apps and connected devices, individuals are now monitoring many of their own personal health indicators. There are activity trackers, such as the Fitbit and Apple Watch, that track steps, distance traveled, and heart rate. There are mattresses that monitor your sleep movement and body temperature. Scales now connect directly to an app to record weight and body fat percentage over time. The apps will usually provide charts to show trends, make recommendations to improve, and even provide reminders. While the data is currently only being used by the individual (well, and the app company to try and sell you other things!), more doctors and hospitals are thinking about how to incorporate all of this data into assessment and treatment programs. While reliability and privacy are still concerns, personal electronic devices are a great way to get individuals more engaged in their own health care. New apps and devices are constantly being invented that will be able to improve remote patient monitoring.

Telehealth Applications Working Together

While the types of telehealth can all be described independently, rarely are they used entirely separately. For example, RPM data may be sent automatically to a monitoring center, but results or concerns may be discussed either synchronously or asynchronously (telephone call or e-mail) with the patient. Or a doctor may call a patient to discuss test results, while also directing the patient to the online portal for documentation of the results. As technology improves, more cross-functional applications of the types of telehealth will likely emerge. New personal RPM devices will be a large driver of this. By combining types of telehealth, more comprehensive remote care and treatment plans will develop to improve access and quality of care.

Recent Developments in Telehealth

Reading through the previous applications of telehealth, you are probably nodding your head, agreeing that you've either used one of these telecommunication methods with your doctor or know someone who has. Many of these telecommunications technologies are so ingrained in our everyday lives that we no longer consciously think about how we're using it. But new technologies and applications are constantly being developed that can improve our health care system. Some of the improvements are small. For example, hospitals are developing apps for home assistant devices (Amazon Alexa or Google Home) that will answer common medical questions such as medication dosing instructions. But some of the recent developments are big and could radically change how the general public accesses medical care. The most important recent development in telehealth is the ability to reach a licensed physician 24/7/365 and have a virtual consultation, either by voice or video call. These virtual networks are not related to a person's primary care doctor or typical hospital, but the doctors are able to diagnose and treat many common ailments as well as aid in chronic condition management. When the media talks about telehealth or telemedicine programs, this specific benefit is what they are often discussing. It's the natural next step in synchronous telehealth technology.

Some people are resistant or hesitant to try out new telehealth methods. Where their health is concerned, people are understandably more conservative. They prefer to do what they have always done and are comfortable with, even it is more inconvenient or expensive. But while calling a licensed doctor via a virtual network to diagnose pink eye, for example, may seem strange, it is just an extension of the technology we already use in our health care system. It is important to keep in mind that at one point, using a telephone was new. Calling a doctor for test results instead of having a follow-up meeting probably made people uncomfortable at first. The jump to using these new applications is no different. While due diligence is required to ensure everyone is getting appropriate medical care, all of these new ways to manage health can help people stay healthy with less inconvenience and expense. Virtual consultations in particular have the potential to radically change how people think about basic medical care.

CHAPTER 3

Telemedicine versus Telehealth

In the literature on remote health care, references to telemedicine and telehealth abound. But what do these terms really mean? Are they the same thing? Unfortunately, in the world of health care, there is no *Merriam-Webster* dictionary of definitions. This has led to confusion and inconsistency in the application of these terms. To attempt to clarify them, many health care organizations have created their own definitions. But some organizations use them interchangeably, while others make important distinctions between the two. The definitions have changed over time, and as technology expands, so does the meaning of the terms "telehealth" and "telemedicine." There have even been new terms, such as "eHealth," that have emerged. There may not be exact consensus yet, but there at least are some general guidelines to help you understand what someone means when he or she uses these terms. We will also explain how this book will use and view these important terms.

History of the Words "Telemedicine" and "Telehealth"

The prefix "tele-" means "far off" or "at a distance." "Medicine" means substances or surgeries used to treat illnesses and disease. "Health" means general soundness of body and mind. Putting these definitions together gives clues into the differences between telemedicine and telehealth, but they don't give the full picture as to how they are used today. To better understand the distinctions between these terms, we first need to look at the history of how these terms developed.

Telemedicine is the older and more widely used of the two terms. It can be found in published literature since the early 1900s as an umbrella term for "delivering remote care." While the idea of remote care had emerged, actual application of telemedicine didn't start until much later because of the limitations of the existing telecommunications technology. Telecommunications technology continued to improve, but it was expensive and required a lot of equipment and expertise. Because of the high investment needed to implement the technology for telemedicine programs, the government was behind many of the first use cases. Starting in the 1960s, the government began to sponsor the first widespread telemedicine projects. These projects focused on providing care to war zones, remote scientific facilities, Native American reservations, and astronauts in space. With the government's help, these organizations were able to invest in the clunky machinery and expensive technology needed to use telemedicine.

As technology improved, the use of telemedicine grew, and the word "telemedicine" became better known. Hospitals started investing in telemedicine equipment to better serve their patients. Still, the equipment was bulky and costly, plus it required trained technicians to use it properly. It was mainly used to transmit data, such as radiology images. The general public had no access to this technology. The first major development in *consumer* use of telemedicine was the telephone. With the rise of the telephone, the public could call their local doctor or hospital for questions and advice. Doctors could also call other specialists when they wanted another opinion. The telephone connected the medical community and their patients. However, consumer telemedicine was still limited to live phone conversations. For any other telemedicine uses, such as transmitting images, patients still had to be at a hospital with the necessary equipment.

The recent advances in telecommunications technology and the invention of the Internet has dramatically changed the telemedicine industry. The average consumer now has broad access to e-mail, videoconferencing, and mobile phones. There are wearable devices that can transmit data directly to either to the wearer or a third party. Hospitals and doctors have patient portals that store patient health information and provide test results. The Internet allows a patient to research a medication or condition before a visit, allowing them to ask better questions—or self-diagnose. Hospitals are developing apps for in-home voice assistants (such as Amazon Alexa or Google Home) that will give dosing instructions for certain medicine. New apps and devices are constantly being developed that expand how the medical community and patients communicate and interact.

Those early uses of telemedicine were narrow compared to the range of services and communication available now. They focused on transmitting medical data or providing a remote physician consultation. It enabled the practice of medicine—hence the word "telemedicine." But new technology has broadened how the public is interacting with the medical community. It no longer simply enables the remote practice of medicine, but it also allows patients to better manage their overall health—hence the emergence of the word "telehealth."

With the rise of this new term, distinctions between the two have attempted to be made. "Telemedicine" now typically refers specifically to using telecommunication technologies such as video, phone calls, and e-mail to support the delivery of physician-provided medical services. "Telehealth," on the other hand, refers to the broader range of healthcare services that can be provided remotely by doctors, nurses, pharmacists, social workers, and health care companies. Just as "health care" no longer refers just to services provided by doctors, "telehealth" encompasses a wide range of services that make up our entire health and wellness experience. This is why the word "telehealth" has grown in popularity in recent years. There is an increasing recognition that our health care system cannot just focus on acute, fee-based care. Instead, we need to focus on quality- and outcomes-based care that helps manage patient and population health. It is no longer just about medicine—it is about health. The current view is that there is a need to prevent health issues, not just treat them. The word "telehealth" recognizes this change in how we view our medical or health care system.

Formal Definitions

Unfortunately, there are no formal definitions for these two terms. But as interest in and applications of these technologies and solutions grows, health care organizations have attempted to define and separate them for the populace to understand. Still, each organization uses them slightly differently, and many have even changed their stances on the terms over time. For example, in recent years, most organizations have decided to use the terms interchangeably or have switched to favoring the term "telehealth" for the reasons described before. To illustrate how these terms have been defined by different organizations over the years, here are examples of their formal definitions or explanations.

The World Health Organization was the first to attempt to define these two terms. In their 2010 report on telemedicine, they studied 104 peer-reviewed definitions of the terms to develop their own comprehensive meaning. The result was this definition of telemedicine: "The delivery of health care services, where distance is a critical factor, by all health care professionals using information and communication technologies for the exchange of vital information for diagnosis, treatment and prevention of disease and injuries, research and evaluation, and for the continuing education of health care providers, all in the interests of advancing the health of individuals and their communities."[6] The report further separated telemedicine and telehealth. Telemedicine was restricted to care delivered only by physicians, whereas telehealth referred to care by any health care professional. However, since that report, the World Health Organization has decided to use the terms interchangeably. The current definition has been simplified but still allows for a widely encompassing range of services: "Telehealth involves the use of telecommunications and virtual technology to deliver health care outside of traditional health care facilities."[7]

In the United States, the US Department of Health and Human Services used to differentiate the two, similarly to the World Health Organization. Telemedicine was considered to be the delivery of remote clinical care. Telehealth was the remote delivery of both clinical and nonclinical care. However, they too have switched to one definition in recent years. They now prefer the term telehealth, meaning "the use of electronic information and telecommunications technologies to support and promote long-distance clinical health care, patient and professional health related education, public health and health administration. Technologies include videoconferencing, the Internet, store-and-forward imaging, streaming media, and terrestrial and wireless communications".

Even the American Telemedicine Association (ATA) uses the two terms interchangeably. Their FAQs state the following: "While some have parsed out unique definitions for each word, ATA treats 'telemedicine' and 'telehealth' as synonyms and uses the terms interchangeably. In both cases, we are referring to the use of remote health care technology to deliver clinical services."[8] Note here that the ATA specifies clinical services. So even though they use the word "telehealth," their meaning is more similar to how other organizations use the word "telemedicine." This is why understanding how a specific company or organization defines the terms can be so important.

Some state departments even craft their own definitions for state policy. For example, California defines telehealth as "the mode of delivering health care services and public health via information and communication technologies to facilitate the diagnosis, consultation, treatment, education, care management, and self-management of a patient's health care while the patient is at the originating site and the health care provider is at a distant site. Telehealth facilitates patient self-management and caregiver support for patients and includes synchronous interactions and asynchronous store and forward transfers."[9] This definition clearly encompasses clinical and nonclinical care.

Other Terms

You may encounter other terms when reading about telehealth. These include eHealth, mHealth, and telecare, among others. Again, every organization and company will use these terms slightly differently. In most cases, the individual has to interpret exactly what these terms mean. Here, however, are some basic definitions.

eHealth is short for "electronic health," just like the words e-mail and e-commerce. It generally encompasses all health care communication and information accessed over the Internet. Examples include everything from a hospital's patient portal that delivers test results to websites such as WebMD, which has a wealth of health information for the public to access.

Similarly, mHealth is short for "mobile health." Any health care delivered via a mobile device could fall under this category. The American Telemedicine Association defines mHealth as "a form of telemedicine using wireless devices and cell phone technologies. It is useful to think of mHealth as a tool—a medium—through which telemedicine can be practiced."[10] Clearly, with the popularity of smart phones, much of eHealth could also be considered mHealth.

The term "telecare" is more frequently used in Europe and the United Kingdom than in the United States. It refers to in-home health care and medical technology that consumers use to monitor their own health. It can include fitness tracking devices, medication reminder systems, or sensors that connect a person directly with medical personnel in an emergency. Telecare is often used in conjunction with telehealth to enable consumers to collect data that helps in remote communications with health care providers.

Our Conclusions

Every article, every organization, and every company may use the words telemedicine and telehealth differently. Until consensus is reached, it's up to the individual to ensure he or she understands how the terms are being used in a specific context. We recommend when reading other literature on the topic or talking to a health care professional that you try and uncover exactly what is meant by the terms. Are they differentiating between the two or are they being used interchangeably? Do they consider nonclinical care to be part of the program? While it may not always matter, the nuances between these terms can help you gain insight into how the organization views remote care. They may focus on remote, clinical diagnoses and treatments. Or they may be referencing a multitude of health and wellness services using telecommunications technology. One is neither better nor worse than the other, but knowing that there can be a difference may help you find the solution and care that you are looking for.

In this book, we will mainly use the word "telehealth," with isolated references to telemedicine when talking about the technology involved. We view telehealth as the wide range of clinical and nonclinical services provided in delivering remote care. We are attempting to be consistent with the general direction of the current literature, while recognizing, as we have demonstrated, that there is no one accepted definition for these terms.

CHAPTER 4

THE PROMISE OF TELEHEALTH

Health care needs an overhaul. It's too expensive and too inconvenient. People are frustrated and dissatisfied with their options, and it doesn't seem like there is anything they can do to have a better experience. And employers, faced with ever-increasing health care costs, are forced to cut benefits and shift costs to employees. But there is a solution out there that can revolutionize how people think about medical care—telehealth.

Telehealth solutions allow employees to have virtual doctor visits. It can make health care cheaper, faster, and easier. Imagine that instead of spending hours and hundreds of dollars at in-person visits, a person could just pick up the phone and speak to a doctor. In minutes, the patient could have a diagnosis, treatment plan, and even a prescription if necessary.

At one time, telehealth seemed like a futuristic dream. But recent technological improvements mean that widespread telehealth can be a reality. More people have smartphones and tablets, there's better cellular networks, and more Wi-Fi hotspots, meaning that anyone, anywhere can now access a doctor at any time of day. Technology has revolutionized other traditional industries, making it more consumer friendly. There's Uber, self-checkout at the grocery store, and now, telehealth consultations.

Helps Individuals

What typically happens when you're sick? You wake up not feeling well, so you call your boss to let him or her know you won't be in today. It's a busy time at work, so you're stressed to be feeling so poorly. You still have your computer, though, so you plan to respond to e-mails and join a few conference calls. You'll do as much work as you can even though you aren't in the office. Next, you call your primary care doctor. Your doctor doesn't have any availability until next week, so your next option is the urgent care center. You head there after responding to a few e-mails, but there are already a few people in the waiting room. The office manager hands you some paperwork, and you sit down to wait. And wait some more. Over an hour later, the doctor finally sees you. He prescribes rest, relaxation, and an antibiotic prescription. You go to a pharmacy to have it filled, and three hours later you're finally home. You missed your meetings and have a backlog of e-mails waiting in your inbox. Not exactly what the doctor ordered. A few weeks later, you get the medical bill, and it's almost $200.

Or what if you're a family with kids? When one of them wakes up with pinkeye, you and your spouse may have to compare schedules to see who is better able to take time off to go to the doctor. Or maybe you argue about whose turn it is to stay home. Then you have to take your sick child to a waiting room filled with other sick children and adults. These difficulties are even more challenging if you're a single parent.

Many of the illnesses we get are the same: colds, flus, a sore throat, earaches, eye infections, and mysterious rashes. These are some of the primary reasons we go to see a doctor or urgent care, yet these are often easily diagnosable using virtual consultations. And going to the doctor isn't cheap. Seeing a primary care doctor for one of these conditions ends up costing $100 on average. If you have to go an urgent care, that number jumps to $160. If an emergency room is necessary, you could be walking away with a whopping bill of over $750. Not to mention the hours spent in the waiting room, the missed work, and the stress caused by the inconveniences.

Getting quality medical care shouldn't be that difficult. Paying $750 to diagnose and get a prescription for pinkeye doesn't make sense. Neither does spending hours in an uncomfortable, germ-filled waiting room. Unfortunately, people think that they don't have a choice. But telehealth can completely change how you access medical care for these common non-emergency illnesses. With virtual consultations, you can speak to a licensed doctor via phone or video in minutes. The telehealth provider ensures that all physicians are highly qualified and specially trained to conduct virtual appointments. They'll review existing medical documents, ask all of the right questions, and make you feel at ease. They'll diagnose and recommend treatment. They can even send prescriptions directly to your regular pharmacy. There's no time limit and no time slots, so you'll never feel rushed. You can take your time to make sure all of your questions are answered and you understand their recommendations. All from the comfort of your own home (or office, or on vacation, or wherever you are).

The best part is that, depending on the provider, there are no claims, no co-pays, and no deductibles. It happens entirely outside of your regular health insurance. The only cost is a small monthly premium for unlimited virtual consultations. So even if the recommendation of the physician is to go see a doctor in person, you haven't wasted any money. Just a few minutes of your time to know who to go see next and even the urgency of seeing someone in person. Health care costs are often confusing and unknown until you get the bill or to the check-out counter after the visit. But with telehealth, you have peace of mind knowing that there won't be any surprise costs for making a call.

Telehealth can be a life saver for busy people and especially families with children. Once school starts, it may seem like at least one of your children is sick every week. Those doctor and pediatrician visits can really add up! But 65 percent of children's illnesses are diagnosable through telehealth. That's more than three of every five times you take a child to the doctor. They can also be helpful in recognizing emergency versus nonemergency situations. When your child wakes up in the middle of the night complaining of an earache, it's hard to know exactly how much pain he or she is in. Can a visit wait until the morning when you could try to see your regular pediatrician? Or do you need to go the emergency room *right now*? Taking just a few minutes to videoconference with a doctor could save you hundreds of dollars.

You may think there's no such thing as a quick and painless visit to a doctor. But common illnesses don't have to cause you stress. With telehealth, these scenarios could happen completely differently. You could skip the drive and the waiting room and be speaking to a doctor in just minutes. Think about what you could do with all of that time back. If the illness is for a family member or is minor, you could save your sick time for a more severe illness. If you're an hourly worker, it could literally mean more money in your pocket. Or you could spend that time resting, sleeping, and recovering instead of stressing about finding an appointment and getting there.

Telehealth is the solution for making medical care easier for common illnesses. There's no reason to waste your valuable time and money when you could be calling a doctor for a fraction of the price and time.

A Solution for Employers

Employers are struggling to provide quality employee benefits at an affordable price. The cost to insure their employees keeps rising, and switching to self-insured and high-deductible health plans can only do so much. Their employees are stressed out, and these changes that reduce the up-front employee benefits cost are hurting productivity and morale. The 2016 Aflac Workforces Report shows that 65 percent of employees have less than $1,000 to pay out-of-pocket expenses for an unexpected illness and 25 percent have had trouble paying a medical bill.[11] And no surprise, employees who are satisfied with their benefits are less likely to have been distracted by a personal issue at work.

Luckily, there is a solution out there that increases employee satisfaction *and* reduces employer health care costs. Telehealth can transform how a workplace thinks about health care. It's a valuable benefit to employees that they care about and will actually use (given the right provider). It saves employee time and increases productivity. It reduces the financial and time stresses that busy employees and families feel when faced with an illness. It can increase employee health and well-being. And best of all, it actually saves employers money. That's right—it's a benefit that directly generates a positive return on investment in *the very first year*.

Right now, your employees are stuck when it comes to medical care. They have to muddle through a system that is confusing, costly, and time consuming. Understanding and accessing care is taking hours out of their work days. When you implement a telehealth solution and educate employees on how to use it, a new world opens up for them. Instead of missing work to take their child to an urgent care for a stomachache or taking a long lunch to get a rash diagnosed, employees can easily have a virtual consultation, via phone or video, and have a diagnosis and treatment plan in just minutes. They can do it at home, before work, or from a private meeting room or office during the day. Instead of hours, getting the care they need will take mere minutes.

Even better, every time they decide to call a doctor instead of heading to a primary care, urgent care, or emergency room, you save money. With many telehealth solutions, the only price is a small per-employee-per-month fee. Then every consultation is free for the patient *and* the employer. That is why a telehealth solution should be able to provide a positive ROI within the first year of implementation.

Too often, employers are forced to choose between lowering their health care costs and providing a great employee benefits package. And while there are other valuable solutions out there, like on-site clinics and wellness programs, none but telehealth guarantees a positive ROI in your first year. And there isn't even a large up-front investment of time and money.

The American Medical Association estimates that telehealth could replace 60–75 percent of doctor office visits and 40–65 percent of emergency room visits.[12] Imagine what those time and money savings could do for your company and your employees.

The Reality of Telehealth Today

Employees and their families get sick every day. So many of these illnesses cause unnecessary stress due to the time, money, and energy spent navigating the current health care system. With telehealth, employees can pick up the phone and have a virtual call with a doctor within minutes. It provides unlimited calls for only a small monthly fee. Technology has changed almost every industry to make it more consumer friendly. Health care is next with telehealth. It's the way of the future.

You may be wondering, if the solution is so great, why you haven't heard more about it. You may even have a telehealth solution already, but you've either never used it, or you're an employer, and you know your employees aren't using it. Unfortunately, many telehealth solutions are not living up to their promise. Average utilization for most solutions is around 7 percent. Telehealth solutions embedded in a major health insurance plan fare even worse with average utilization rates at 1 percent. These solutions often have co-pays that deter use. And the providers are not effectively communicating with employees about how and why to use the benefit. Employee benefits brokers are not helping, either. Most know nothing about telehealth solutions. If they even suggest it to an employer, they don't know enough to help pick an effective solution.

The truth is, there is a solution out there that can help people and employers with their health care. And hopefully this book can shed some light on why it's being hidden and how to find a solution that will actually work for you.

CHAPTER 5

Why Aren't Brokers Selling Telehealth?

The natural place for the sale of telehealth solutions is through an employee benefits broker. Companies hire brokers to help them design and implement employee benefits plans. It seems like it should be straightforward. Brokers learn about the value of telehealth solutions through industry news, events, and colleagues. Or telehealth companies go to a broker's office to tell them directly about their solutions. They'd be wowed at the potential savings and the addition of a meaningful benefit to employees. Then the broker would take the solution to clients as part of their overall employee benefits plans and strategies. But the slow adoption of telehealth shows that this isn't happening. Unfortunately, many brokers simply do not find it worth the time and effort to learn about and sell telehealth programs. To understand why, we first have to understand how most brokers make their money.

Benefits Brokers: The Basics

The very basic function of an employee benefits broker is to match insurance carriers to companies. A company with an employee benefits plan or that wants to implement one will hire a broker to reach out to insurance companies for bids. The broker will negotiate with the insurance companies, present the bids to the employer, and provide a recommendation. Once the employer chooses providers, the broker will also help implement and manage the benefits program. Types of insurance include health, vision, dental, life, and disability. Each year when the insurance companies issue their price per member for the annual renewal of benefits, called premiums, the broker will present the premiums to the employer. If the price is too high, the broker may negotiate with the incumbent provider or go back out to bid to multiple insurance companies.

Most benefits brokers, however, have evolved to also function as advisers and consultants. Companies will share their strategic goals, both financial and HR-related, and the broker will work to see how the employee benefits package can help the company achieve those goals. The right employee benefits package can help an employer reduce costs, improve employee retention, or attract top executive talent. Brokers can recommend tweaking medical plan offerings, bumping up the disability insurance or adding a new wellness benefit. Employers rely on their brokers to be knowledgeable and informed on all aspects of benefits and benefits management, including regulatory compliance.

With the passage of the Affordable Care Act came many changes to health care, including changes to employer requirements. Employers often trust their brokers to understand the current regulatory environment and to ensure that their plans meet all the requirements. There can be hefty fines if an employer doesn't meet the government regulations or time lines.

Employers place a lot of trust in their brokers to build them the best employee benefits plan and to help them navigate the complexities of the regulatory requirements. But employee benefits brokers are not considered fiduciaries, meaning that brokers are not required to place their client's interests above their own. This is important to keep in mind when dealing with an employee benefits broker. And when you understand how most brokers make their money, it helps explain why they are not bringing telehealth solutions to their clients.

Employee benefits brokers typically make their money in one of two ways: fees or commissions, although the majority are commission based. With a fee-based broker, the employer will pay the broker either a flat fee or hourly rate for his or her work. With a commission-based broker, the *insurance companies* pay the broker a small percentage of the total premium paid by employers who select their products. This commission is built into the cost employers, and individuals are paying for their insurance. For example, if the employer is paying $100,000 a year to the health insurance company for its employees and health insurance plans and the broker's commission rate is 6 percent, the broker will make $6,000 on that plan. Many brokers also get kickbacks from insurance companies for selling a certain amount of their products. As an example, if a broker sells $1 million worth of the insurance company's health plan, the broker may get an additional $10,000 kickback in addition to the commission percentage of each sale.

As you can imagine, this places the broker in a conflict of interest with his or her clients. Employers want as low of premiums as possible. But the more premium the employer pays, the more money the broker makes. And the kickbacks may induce a broker to recommend one insurance company over another if their kickbacks are better, even if it is not in the best interest of the client to choose that provider. Many brokers work almost exclusively with a handful of insurance companies. They may say they work with everyone, but in practice 90 percent of their business goes to the same insurance companies.

Many laws and regulations have cracked down on these practices in recent years, but the truth is it still happens. So while employers are putting all of their faith in their broker to provide the best advice, solutions, and recommendations, that is not what is happening in reality. Brokers are putting their interests above those of their clients, meaning their goal is to make the most money, not to provide the best service. To make the most money, brokers do whatever they can to attract and retain clients while maximizing profit for the amount of time invested. It is a balancing act between providing good enough service to clients to keep them without doing so much that it reduces their profit margins.

"Not Worth My Time"

One of the consequences of a commission-based business is that brokers tend to spend the majority of their time and energy on the expensive products, such as health insurance plans. A telehealth solution, compared to health insurance, is extremely inexpensive. So, in most instances, a broker makes much less money implementing a telehealth solution compared to a health insurance plan. To make matters worse, telehealth can be just as time consuming to sell and implement as health insurance.

When you consider that the brokers, employers, and employees often aren't well educated on telehealth solutions, it takes a lot of up-front time investment from the broker to learn about telehealth. Then they have to educate their clients and convince them that it's worth their time and money too. Even if they convince an employer to implement a solution, they may then have to work closely with the employer to educate their employees about telehealth. In consulting, where time is money, brokers prefer to spend this time on other, more profitable activities.

Employers also want to spend most of their time with their brokers talking about the health insurance plan. For many employers, health insurance is their second-biggest expense. And health care costs have increased faster than economic productivity has increased, which means that health insurance costs are taking a bigger percentage of company earnings. In a study by Willis Towers Watson, health care costs as a percentage of employee pay increased from 5.7 percent to 11.5 percent from 2001 to 2015.[13] That's almost double, and companies aren't expecting the trend to stop any time soon. This is obviously a concern to many employers. In the Wells Fargo Employee Benefits Strategies, Actions, and Behaviors Study from 2016, the number-one HR concern for the short *and* long term is managing the overall cost of health care benefits.[14] So when employers are talking to their brokers, their focus is also mainly on the health insurance plan. But the brokers have tunnel vision when it comes to reducing health care costs. Instead of trying to be creative and offer new, proven solutions, brokers are doing what they've always done to reduce costs: changing the health care plan offerings or the provider.

Every year, a company's incumbent health insurance provider will issue their renewal—the per-employee premium to keep the same plan as the previous year. If the renewal price is too high, the company's broker will either try to negotiate with the provider or will look to other health insurance providers to see what they would charge. If the costs are still too high for the employer, the broker will help the company look at different plan designs. Sometimes they'll offer a less rich benefit with higher co-pays. Or maybe they'll switch to a high deductible health plan (HDHP) format. Some employers limit spousal health care coverage. Most of the "solutions" using this strategy simply shift more of the costs from the employer to the employee. Even if these strategies keep employee premiums lower, the change in plan designs ensure that the employee is paying more of the total medical costs. The truth is in the financials: in 2000, patient payments only accounted for 5 percent of health care provider revenue. In 2017, this number has risen dramatically to 35 percent of revenue. It's proof that these strategies do almost nothing to reduce total health care costs—they just help the employers meet their financial targets. But if the broker doesn't present other solutions, the employers feel like their back is up against the wall. They have to cut benefits even if they don't want to.

Employers trust their brokers to be the experts. So even though the broker isn't really helping solve the problem, the client may still be satisfied, thinking that the broker is doing the best he or she can.

Workplace Wellness

Some brokers get slightly more creative with their solutions. Maybe they're a bigger brokerage, or maybe the employer has pressured them to bring other ideas to the table. In these instances, a broker normally turns to a wellness solution. Wellness as a concept has grown rapidly in the consumer market, and it has penetrated all the way to workplace solutions. "Wellness" has become a buzzword in the employee benefits space. Since many people spend the majority of their day at work, they are asking their employers for help and solutions to improve workplace wellness. In turn, the employers are turning to their brokers to find them a solution.

Workplace wellness solutions not only fulfill an employee demand, but they also promise to actually reduce health care costs in the long term by improving employee health. It's very appealing to an employer. The Affordable Care Act also put in place new incentives that promote employer wellness programs. Based on these demands and market conditions, brokers are sometimes bringing wellness solution ideas to employers as a way to reduce costs. Unfortunately, these programs are not yet proven as a way to reduce costs. There is a lot of skepticism over the ROI claims of many wellness companies. And any results are usually seen in the long term, not immediately. But employees are jumping on the wellness bandwagon, so employers and brokers are bringing them what they ask for.

Demand More

Ideally, a company's benefits broker would be knowledgeable about every possible benefits program, and they would present strategic plans and options to their clients using a mix of solutions. But that is not how most brokers are operating today. Instead, they are simply reacting to employer's requests to cut up-front costs from their health insurance premiums or to implement a wellness program. This is enough to keep their clients happy, their commissions high, and their workload low. But innovation is being left behind, and there are other solutions, such as telehealth, that are getting overlooked.

A good telehealth solution is guaranteed to provide positive ROI to the employer in the *first* year. Changing your plan design or workplace wellness programs can't deliver on promises like that. Plan design changes simply shift the burden to employees. Workplace wellness may indeed work, but it's not going to work as quickly as a telehealth solution. Employers and employees need savings now, not in five years. But brokers don't have a good financial incentive to deliver on innovation. After all, the brokers get paid a percentage of total premium, so the higher the premiums, the more they make. Brokers' true incentives are to do enough to help their clients reduce costs to keep them happy and to keep them as clients without actually coming up with a solution that lowers their clients' costs.

But employees and employers need to demand more from their employee benefits brokers. There are creative solutions and programs out there that can reduce costs and provide a meaningful benefit to your employees. Brokers should be the ones researching the options and presenting ideas to achieve their clients' strategic goals. They are failing in their task of helping employers best manage their plans. If you're an employer, it's time to examine what your broker is really doing for you. Most benefits brokers simply are not putting their clients' interests first. Their number-one focus is their own profit, and employers and employees are suffering because of it.

CHAPTER 6

FINDING A SOLUTION THAT WORKS

Without financial incentives, brokers haven't cared to learn about or understand telehealth. But that isn't to say that no brokers are actually selling it. Most brokers have at least heard of it. Maybe a telehealth company has contacted them or presented to them. Maybe they read about it in the *Wall Street Journal*. Or maybe a client came to them asking about it. But there is a big difference between knowing generally what telehealth is and actually understanding how it works and how to implement it as part of a comprehensive cost-saving strategy. Instead, brokers know just enough to "check the box" on telehealth when a client asks for it.

Because of this, brokers aren't doing their due diligence on researching telehealth. They're selling you ineffective solutions. But there is a solution out there that can save you money. Telehealth could be a game changer for the entire system, but brokers don't care enough to learn about it. They're content to do as little as possible and to sit comfortably on their increasing profits. Telehealth can save you money and increase employee satisfaction and productivity. But how are you supposed to find a solution that actually works?

Is Your Solution Working?

If a broker sells telehealth, it is usually offered by the health insurance company and is embedded in the health insurance plan. It seems like a "free" benefit for employers to offer their employees. And the broker gets to seem innovative to clients and make more money without doing much additional work. But if brokers really understood telehealth, they would know that these add-on programs are ineffective and the costs are either passed on to the employees or are built into the regular premiums. Often the health insurance company increases their premiums to offer telehealth, so the broker gets more money for little effort. Once the employer buys in, however, the broker stops thinking about it. They never check to see if the added benefit is actually working for the employer.

If you have a telehealth solution, have you ever seen a utilization report? Utilization is the most important number to know about a telehealth solution. It reflects how many employees are actually using the benefit. If you're paying for a benefit that no one is using, you're throwing money down the drain. But most brokers never run utilization reports. If the employer doesn't ask for them, why bother? And the sad truth is that for most solutions bundled with the health insurance, the utilization is really low—about 1–3 percent. No broker wants to show that kind of number to a client.

This isn't just a problem with small brokerages. I once went into a nationally known brokerage to talk to them about my telehealth solution. They were currently selling telehealth to their clients with their health insurance. So, I asked them, "Have you ever run a utilization report?" They hadn't. Why? They said, "Our clients are happy." To them, as long as employers aren't complaining, they're going to stick with the status quo. They do not care if your employee benefits are working, as long as you're happy and keep using them as a broker. So, they'll happily sell you a solution that masquerades as a cost-saving technique, even though it just makes their and the insurance companies' wallets fatter.

To get around this, I often try selling directly to employers. My numbers speak for themselves, and many employers want to use my solution once they speak with me. But the brokers don't feel like doing more work for a client that's not asking for anything. I was working with a broker once, and he just wasn't interested in bringing my solution to clients. His clients were happy, and he didn't see any need to bring in a new solution. So, I went directly to one of his clients and talked to them about my solution. I showed them the numbers and explained to them how much it would help the business and the employees, and they were sold. When the broker found out, he was furious. He wanted to make his commission, even though he didn't do the work. I told him too bad, and his response was that he would *never* work with me again or bring me in front of any of his clients. So, unless I go directly to his other clients, those employers will never know about the possibilities available with my solution. Is your broker doing that to you? These are the people who say that they're bringing employers the best cost-saving solutions out there. But we know that isn't true.

What Brokers *Should* Be Looking For

Not all telehealth solutions are equal. Brokers should be critically evaluating all of the telehealth solutions available to determine what works best for their clients. A good telehealth solution can provide a meaningful benefit to employees *and* save employers money.

First, brokers need to look at each solution's utilization and participation rates. These are the two most important metrics, and as an employer, you shouldn't pick a solution until you know how these metrics compare across competitors. The utilization rate is the number of consultations per eligible employees. It indicates how frequently the solution is being used. The higher the rate, the more benefit you and your employees are getting out of the solution. Many solutions bundled with health insurance have average utilization rates around 3 percent. A good solution should have average rates at 30 percent or above. Make sure your broker is probing for details on this metric. Each provider should have calculated this number the same way. You may want to see their highest and lowest utilization rate from the past year or the average utilization rate of first-year clients.

The participation rate is the number of consultations from *unique employees* per eligible employees. This number shows how widespread adoption of the benefit is. Utilization could be skewed by a subset of employees heavily using the benefit.

But the participation rate will show how popular the benefit is among all employees. A solution with consistently high participation rates probably has a strong communication strategy that enables them to engage with more employees. A good rule of thumb is the participation rate should be about half of the utilization rate. A strong participation rate is critical to ensuring that your solution is successful. You'll see the largest increases in employee satisfaction and productivity if more people are aware of and use the benefit.

Second, brokers should examine the implementation and engagement process of each solution. For many employers and employees, telehealth is a new way to access medical care. But changing people's health care habits isn't easy. That's why it's crucial to partner with a provider who delivers a thorough onboarding and communication program. This helps ensure high utilization and participation rates. Employers shouldn't be in charge of implementing a telehealth solution. HR teams are not the experts on telehealth; the telehealth provider is. The provider should work with your HR team to develop a comprehensive employee communication and engagement plan. Some companies only offer generic brochures that you can mail or e-mail to employees. Or they'll leave the implementation work to the broker. But the broker doesn't care if your employees are actually using telehealth. If they've sold it to you, they've already made their money. But with such a new benefit, a canned e-mail isn't enough to actually engage your employees. Virtual medical visits are new and confusing. Employees will have a lot of questions. You need a plan tailored to your employee demographic that includes multiple deliveries and forms of communications to reach the broadest number of employees. Otherwise, they will disregard the benefit and continue to access medical care the way they already have.

Third, brokers should compare solutions' expected and average return on investment (ROI) for employers. Telehealth should always be able to generate a positive ROI. When comparing ROI claims, look closely at the calculations. They should be straightforward, based on savings from diverted costs of in-person visits due to telemedicine. No other costs "savings," such as productivity gains, should be included. While these are real benefits, a telehealth solution should be able to directly pay for itself through diverted health care costs. In addition to their ROI estimates, providers should also show the ROI for their other clients to confirm it's consistently positive. Since ROI is so important for most companies, look for a provider that will guarantee a positive ROI in the contract. When you select a provider that holds themselves accountable for financial results, you are choosing a provider whose interests align with the employer's.

Fourth, brokers need to understand the total cost of the solution. Not all telehealth solutions are set up the same way. Most providers charge a per-employee-per-month (PEPM) fee, which can range anywhere from fifty cents to fifteen dollars. However, the providers with the lowest PEPM price often charge an additional fee per consultation, paid by the employee, that can be anywhere from twenty to fifty dollars per call. To employers and brokers, this may seem great because it lowers their cost. But these solutions typically have low ROI and utilization rates. The consultation fee is a barrier that discourages employee utilization. So the up-front cost may be lower, but the employer won't actually save any money by diverting costs from expensive sites of care to a virtual consultation. In addition to the PEPM price, some providers will charge additional hidden fees. There can be fees for onboarding, communication plans, and even excess utilization fees. Employers and brokers needs to read all contracts closely to ensure there are no hidden surprises when it comes time to pay the provider. The best solutions should have no additional fees for the employer or employees besides the PEPM charge.

Fifth, brokers should evaluate the user experience. Underlying all of the rate, pricing, and implementation concerns, the solution needs to deliver a valuable benefit and an outstanding user experience. The solution should enable easy sign up and the ability to place a call in the same day. Employees should have a short waiting time to be able to talk directly with a licensed physician who can write prescriptions. The service should be available in all states, every day, at all hours. All consultations should be reviewed and recorded for quality assurance. At the end of the day, a solution that employees like to use is what makes telehealth a meaningful benefit. It's what saves an employer money and creates value for employees.

Employers Beware

When it comes to telehealth, brokers aren't doing their job. When I go into a brokerage to talk about a solution, my first question is always, "Do you sell telehealth solutions to your clients?" The response is almost always the same. People look around the room, hoping someone else knows. Someone finally mumbles that they think they do, but it's bundled with their health insurance. No one knows how much they sell or if the solutions are working for their clients. No one pays any attention to it. And even when I present my arguments and my numbers, many of them just don't care.

If you think your broker is bringing you all the solutions available, think again. Brokers are trying to do as little work as possible to keep you happy. And if you have a telehealth solution, ask them to look at the numbers. They probably aren't good. Brokers could be bringing clients a game-changing solution, but they're only looking out for themselves and their own wallets. Employer and employee health care costs *can* be lower. There are options out there. Brokers are just choosing to ignore them.

CHAPTER 7

Health Insurance Companies and Their Telehealth Solutions

When telehealth companies offering virtual consultations first emerged, health insurance companies didn't know how to react. But quickly, they began to see these telehealth companies as an opportunity instead of competition. The major health insurance carriers and the big telehealth companies began a partnership. The health insurer will package the telehealth solution with its health insurance, making them more money *and* appearing to be innovative. For the big telehealth companies, they got access to the health insurers' existing customers, which equaled rapid growth. It's a win-win for these two markets. Unfortunately, it's a losing scenario for the people who could actually benefit from telehealth.

At first, it may seem like it should be a win for people and employees as well. They get access to a new, useful benefit that's already packaged into their existing health plan, often subsidized by their employer. What's the problem? The problem is that the health insurance companies care about maximizing profit, not about making health care more accessible and affordable. And they make more money by *not* educating people about telehealth. You read that correctly. They're selling you a solution that they don't care if people know about or use. They've decided that marketing telehealth is more expensive than it's worth, and so they just won't spend the money. The only reason they're providing the solution in the first place is to appear innovative to their clients. Employees and employers are the ones who suffer because they are missing out on a solution that has the potential to be a complete game changer for medical care.

How Insurance Companies' Telehealth Solutions Operate

The payment structure of embedded telehealth solutions is long and complex. After all, in between the employees and the actual telehealth provider, there are the employers, the brokers, and the health insurance company. Each level contributes to the complexity in the cost structure and the dilution of the effectiveness of the solution.

First, the insurance company will pay a small per-employee-per-month (PEPM) fee, anywhere from fifteen to twenty cents, to the telehealth company. This extra cost is built into the monthly health insurance premium that the employer pays. Then, the broker takes a percentage of the total premium as commission. Additionally, the employee will have a co-pay, or consultation fee, for each virtual visit, which can be anywhere from twenty to sixty dollars. Some employers cover this cost. The consultation fee is typically split between the insurance company and the telehealth company.

On the surface, it seems like the insurance company and the telehealth company would want more employees to use the solution. After all, they get the consultation fee each time someone uses it. Unfortunately, the health insurance companies have not figured out how to effectively market telehealth. It would cost more for them to educate and engage employees than they would see returned in utilization fees.

Insurance companies only care about profit. They do not care about educating patients or employers, patient health, or improving access to care. They underwrite based on the current system and population risk and then charge accordingly. The real incentive for a health insurance carrier to provide telehealth is the appearance of innovation without doing any work. That's why many insurance providers rebrand a third-party telehealth solution to make it seem like their own system. Telehealth is a shiny new object that they can point to when talking to employers about why to choose them, even though they know that it won't end up benefiting the employer or employees. It's merely for appearances. That's why they don't bother to encourage utilization or provide a great user experience.

To the employer and employees, the health insurance companies sell the telehealth solution as a free solution. But don't be fooled. Any cost they incur in providing the solution is built into the employer and employee premiums. The health insurance premiums build in all operational costs, including telehealth. And what's the point of a "free" benefit if no one is using it?

They Don't Care If People Use It

Since the cost of marketing telehealth is greater than the potential return, insurance companies spend as little money as possible on the telehealth solutions. They don't put many resources toward communication *or* the solution. The result is low utilization and a terrible user experience. The insurance companies simply don't care whether people use the solution or not.

But with modern psychology and marketing knowledge, we know that changing people's behavior is hard. Virtual consultations are new to the majority of people. To get people to change how they're accessing medical care, there needs to be a complete education and awareness campaign. But telehealth offered by major health insurers usually lacks any robust communication with employees. At most there will be a one-time generic brochure or e-mail to send to employees.

A friend of mine recently got a new job, and with it, new health insurance from one of the major carriers. When she got the introductory packet in the mail, she browsed through it and saw one bullet point about their embedded telehealth solution. It had a phone number you could call or a website address you could go to. That's it. One bullet point in an entire packet that, let's be honest, most people never even look through. After all, she'd already signed up for the plan, so they weren't trying to sell her anything. She probably wouldn't have even noticed if it she hadn't been familiar with telehealth through me. How is that level of communication going to change consumer behavior? Even if someone saw it and was interested, it would probably be forgotten by the time it was actually needed. Ongoing communication is needed so that telehealth is top of mind when someone actually needs medical care.

And even when someone does bother to try to use the bundled telehealth solution, the user experience will likely prevent them from completing the visit or ever using it again. Many of these solutions have a complicated registration process. There may even be a waiting period between registration and when the employee can actually schedule a consultation. Not to mention the long average wait times to speak to the doctor! Then the employee finds out that there's a co-pay *and* possible additional costs from the claim. The whole process seems frustrating. If an employee even completes the process, it's unlikely they'll choose to use it again.

There's more: if, somehow, an employer develops its own telehealth communication strategy and gets employees to use it, many of these bundled solutions have an excess utilization fee in the contract. That means if an employer's utilization goes above a certain number, often 20 percent, the employer will be charged a fee. So even the employer has a disincentive to drive high utilization. They'll be punished for using their "free" solution.

With this combination of poor communication, bad user experience, and disincentives to use the solution, it's no surprise that these solutions don't perform. There's low utilization and awareness that these benefits are even available. To be effective, a telehealth solution needs to have a custom communication strategy with multiple touch points in different formats (print, e-mail) throughout the year. It should answer questions about how, why, and when to use telehealth. Then, the user experience needs to be simple. Employees need to be able to sign up and make a call, with a short wait time, on the same day. There can't be fees or surprise charges to discourage adoption. The solution needs to be top of mind for employees when they need medical attention, and it needs to be a great experience to keep them coming back!

The Real Cost to Employers

Besides getting ripped off by the insurance company's false promises, employers are also missing out on the savings that a good telehealth solution can actually provide. In contrast to bundled telehealth, stand-alone telehealth solutions require an up-front payment from the employer. Instead of the insurance company paying a PEPM fee to the telehealth company, the employer pays the PEPM fee. However, in a good telehealth solution, the *only* cost is the PEPM fee. There are no employee co-pays. No claims are generated for either the employee or employer. And there's definitely no excess utilization fee.

But because there's no payment barrier for employees, these solutions typically get much higher average utilization. The average utilization for carrier-embedded telehealth is 1–3 percent. For a standalone solution, the average could be as high as 37 percent. For self-funded employers, each time an employee chooses to call a virtual provider instead of going to an urgent care or emergency room, the employer saves money. Let's look at an example of how the savings might work for an employer:

For a two-thousand-person self-funded company, an embedded telehealth solution will only eliminate around twenty unnecessary in-person medical visits. This could save the company $12,300 over the course of the year – a nominal amount when you consider the total cost of health care spend for an employer.

If the same company had gone with a stand-alone solution, the savings could be over $500,000. Even with an upfront PEPM fee, which may be somewhere around five dollars, the net savings is substantial, especially when compared to the embedded telehealth solution. This dramatic increase in savings is due directly to the increased utilization that these solutions have. And this figure doesn't even include the productivity savings employers see. Employees that use telehealth will spend less time away from work to see doctors and have less medical financial stress. It directly affects employee effectiveness and focus at work.

We can get this level of utilization by removing the barriers to telehealth. There's no consultation fee, and no claim is generated. Our user experience is easy and fast. We have figured out how to effectively market our solution so that employees will sign up and use it. We're so confident in our solution that we contractually guarantee a positive ROI for our clients. If an employer doesn't see a greater return from diverted health care costs than it cost them to implement our solution, we refund the excess. Employers can't lose when they implement our solution.

Employees Get Screwed

Employers aren't the only ones missing out on savings. With carrier-embedded telehealth, not only does the employee have to pay a co-pay, but the call also generates a claim, just like any in-person visit. And with deductibles for most plans being sky-high, that means the employee will likely pay for a good portion of the visit out of pocket. The virtual visit could end up costing the same or only slightly less than a physician's office visit. This is a huge barrier for employees and embedded telehealth solutions to overcome.

Changing people's behavior is already hard. Even if someone—the employer, the broker, the insurance company, or the telehealth company—were to actually educate and market to the employees, the cost of these solutions will deter most people from utilizing it. Think about it: if you had to pay to use a new service that you were unsure about, would you use it? What if you ended up having to go an in-person doctor anyway, and now you'll have to pay twice?

That's why so many services have free trials. There is a lot of psychological friction to overcome to get people to try something new. If they have to pay before they even try it, most people will just never bother. With medical care, the friction is even stronger because there is more fear of the unknown. Without proper communication, employees often don't understand what is covered and what's not, what the costs are, or what conditions to call in for. With medical care, it doesn't seem worth the risk, so people will continue accessing care the way they always have. And they'll continue to miss out on the financial savings and convenience that telehealth can offer.

That is why it is important to choose a provider that puts the end user first. The company needs to want people to actually *use* the solution. Telehealth has the potential to change how the public thinks about medical care. It's more affordable, more convenient, and less stressful than trying to schedule an in-person visit. For example, for pinkeye the average urgent care cost is $102 and the average emergency room cost is $370. This is easily diagnosable via a virtual visit that is completely free for the employee. Employees are struggling with medical care today, and there is a solution out there that can help them. The insurance companies just don't care if they know about it.

You Get What You Pay For

As with most things in life, with telehealth you get what you pay for. These "free" solutions offered by the major health insurance companies are not really free. They provide no meaningful benefit to the employer or the employees. If you currently have telehealth through your health insurance carrier, look closely to see what the solution is really getting you. There is a telehealth solution out there that can guarantee a positive ROI *and* can make a real difference for employees. But it's not through your health insurance.

CHAPTER 8

WHY YOU SHOULDN'T DUMP TELEHEALTH ON HR

When a company is considering a telehealth benefit, they often turn to their human resources department to handle the implementation and employee communication. After all, HR is in charge of all employee benefits. Unfortunately, this is one of the leading reasons that most companies have really low utilization from their telehealth solution. HR should not be responsible for implementing telehealth. They do not have the motivation, the skills, or the knowledge needed to effectively implement and drive results from the benefit.

The sad truth is that if a company dumps responsibility for telehealth on HR, it will likely become a wasted benefit. Employees will not use it, and many will not even know they have access to the benefit. Instead, companies should choose a provider that assumes responsibility for the success of the solution and does the work itself. Only then will your company and the employees reap all of the benefits telehealth has to offer.

HR Is Sick of Employee Benefits

The human resources department serves as the go-between for employees and company management. They deal with recruiting, hiring, training, payroll, employee-employer disputes, and the employee benefits package. But as employee benefits have gotten more complicated and more contentious, HR has gotten increasingly frustrated with employee benefits as a whole.

Every year, HR professionals everywhere dread employee benefit implementation and open-enrollment season. They get bombarded with questions and complaints from every side. CEOs and CFOs always want to run the numbers. Benefit costs are rising, especially health care costs, and CEOs and CFOs are understandably concerned. They put pressure on HR to reduce costs while still providing an enticing benefits package. That means most years do not involve just a standard renewal of all the employee benefits. Instead, HR is forced to evaluate their current plans to see where there are potential savings. With the employee benefits broker's help, HR will have to see how different plan designs or different providers affect total cost.

Even with a broker's help, this process is still a lot of work for HR. And unfortunately, it's mostly data entry and data pulling. Every possible provider needs an up-to-date employee file, and each one with different information. The retirement plan companies need updated salary information and every spouse's date of birth. The disability provider needs to know every employee's job classification and the company's disability claim history. The list goes on. Computers and sophisticated software should make this process easier, but too often it's the opposite. HR is stuck with multiple systems that do not talk to each other, resulting in repetitive entries of the same information and too much room for error. Someone who retired might be updated in one system but still be listed as an active employee in another. HR might not have the birth date for an employee's new spouse. All of this has to be manually updated and entered. Inevitably, providers come back with questions and discrepancies, each of which has to be looked up and verified to find the right information. It's tedious, time consuming, and let's be honest, *boring*. It's no surprise that HR professionals are sick of employee benefits and dread dealing with it.

To make matters worse, rarely is everyone happy with the end results. HR is the group that has to deal with the aftermath and fallout from any changes. In the current environment, "changes" often mean benefit cuts and cost shifting to employees. Nasty employee complaints are becoming all too common. On the other side, the CEO and CFO do not think the savings are good enough and worry about the bottom line. HR is stuck in the middle, trying to make these two groups happy. Even if benefits have improved or there's a new benefit being added, HR will still have to handle all of the many employee questions and concerns.

So when asked to or tasked with implementing *another* solution, such as telehealth, HR, understandably, usually isn't too thrilled. The last thing they want to deal with is another company asking for employee records, another set of enrollment kits to send out, and one more thing for employees to call or e-mail about with questions or concerns. They simply do not want to implement another solution. Many HR departments will resist adding a benefit, even when the numbers justify it. And if they do end up having to implement it, unless someone is holding them directly accountable for telehealth, their attitude will cause them to drag their feet, make mistakes, and generally do a poor job. It doesn't set up the new solution for success.

HR Is Not Marketing

The number-one reason most telehealth programs fail is because of the marketing strategy, or should I say lack of marketing strategy. The majority of telehealth companies and brokers leave the marketing up to the HR department. But when the communication responsibility is dumped on HR, the solution almost always falls short of expectations. That's why the majority of employees that have access to a solution do not even know that it exists. And if they do know about it, odds are they have not used it. They probably only vaguely know about it, and might not even know where to go for more information. The problem is that HR is not a marketing department. If you give them a generic e-mail to send out to all employees, sure, they'll send it. But that's not enough to drive utilization.

To change employee behavior, a strategic communication plan needs to be developed that is specific to an employer and their employees. Is it a mostly blue-collar manufacturing company with locations throughout the Midwest? Or is it a white-collar startup with just one corporate office and on-the-road salespeople? These two companies will not have the same needs and will not be best reached the same way. For the manufacturing company, one of the biggest draws of telehealth will be the ability to have a doctor's appointment without having to clock out and lose valuable paid hours from your day. For the startup, one communication piece could focus on how helpful telehealth can be when you need medical care while on the road. Companies need enrollment kits in the mail, e-mail blasts, brochures, and posters in break rooms. They need to provide relevant, timely communication that keeps telehealth top of mind when employees need care.

Reading that, does it sound like something most HR teams could develop and implement all on their own? With only a few generic brochures from the provider to start with? Probably not. HR can send out e-mails, resolve employee concerns, and keep payroll straight. What they cannot do is create and execute on a telehealth communication strategy that will drive the utilization your company needs to realize the benefits of telehealth. They are not even experts in telehealth—they need to be educated on the benefit too! How can they be expected to succeed on a topic they have limited to no knowledge of? Especially when they're already sick of employee benefits?

Marketing telehealth is hard. It's a new benefit that asks employees to change the habits they have established around health care. In fact, health insurance companies, brokers, and most telehealth providers do not know how to effectively market telehealth either. That is why they shift the burden to HR. They do not know how to do it themselves, so they want HR to take the blame when the solution does not live up to its promises.

The biggest hurdle for the entire telehealth industry to overcome is low utilization due to poor marketing. That's why companies need to choose a telehealth provider that does the marketing for them. Companies that have figured out how to market telehealth effectively will be able to show prospective clients the numbers that prove their strategy works. The provider should work *with* HR teams to develop a year-long, custom communication plan. Then they should execute on that plan. Not HR. Employees should get multiple touchpoints throughout the year so they know about their benefit, as well as how, why, and when to use it. It's the only way to get an average utilization over 30 percent. When HR is responsible for the marketing of your telehealth solution, you will not get those kinds of results. You need experts that care about the benefit, not an apathetic HR department.

Who Is Accountable for Results?

While HR is often the responsible business unit for overseeing employee benefits, they are not typically held accountable for the results. After all, so much of employee benefit costs are out of their control. Their goals focus on turnover, employee satisfaction, cost per hire, time to fill, and other similar metrics that HR can really influence. But if HR isn't accountable for the results of the employee benefits, including telehealth, who is? Most employers would say their broker is responsible. But we've already established that brokers are not interested in and are not knowledgeable about telehealth. They are not running utilization reports or including telehealth metrics in quarterly reviews. If on the off chance someone does run the report, the bad results probably kept them from sharing it with the employer. They would rather ignore it than address why the solution is not performing. In the rare case that an employer actually asks to see the utilization, brokers will merely blame HR for the poor results.

No one is really accountable for the results of these telehealth solutions, which is why the utilization rates are so low. As with most things, accountability is key to making any new initiative work. Without a specific goal, HR will not do the work necessary to make telehealth a success. But it may be an impossible task. On the one hand, holding HR accountable for the results would likely improve their implementation and communication around telehealth. On the other hand, is it really fair to hold HR accountable for a solution that is not their own and that they know very little about? Not really.

A telehealth provider should assume responsibility for their solution. They should take charge of the marketing and implementation process to maximize utilization. Telehealth companies need to communicate with their clients on their solution. They should provide utilization reports and help clients understand how telehealth is saving the business and the employees time and money. The best part? They need put their money where their mouth is by providing an actual savings guarantee. The solution should save a self-funded company more money than it costs, or they should refund the difference. Hold themselves financially accountable for the results, so companies can be confident that they will take implementation, marketing, and customer service seriously. That is how, your telehealth solution will be a success.

Set Yourself Up for Success

The majority of telehealth solutions are managed by HR teams. The majority of telehealth solutions also have utilization rates around 1 percent. It is not just a coincidence. HR does not want another employee benefit to manage. It's too much work and too much effort. They do not have the skill set or the accountability to make a telehealth solution live up to the promises.

Telehealth works when it is executed correctly. But to do that, employers need to choose a provider that does the work itself instead of shifting the work to the HR team. Unfortunately, most employers who look to implement a telehealth solution will simply choose the cheapest provider. However, a provider that does the marketing and communication itself is not going to be the cheapest. There are obvious additional costs associated with marketing that have to be built into the employer's cost. But by paying slightly more up front, employers can get a solution that actually delivers. Not to mention the savings guarantee that we offer.

If all an employer wants is to check the box on telehealth, they can go ahead and dump all the responsibility on HR. But if an employer wants a solution that can benefit their bottom line and increase employee satisfaction, they need to choose a provider that handles the hard work themselves.

CHAPTER 9

Telehealth Needs Executive Engagement

For telehealth to live up to its full potential, executives, specifically CEOs and CFOs, need to be more involved in the decision making. CEOs and CFOs are busy. They have a lot on their plates, and very rarely, if ever, do they come from an employee benefits background. Their focus is usually on operational efficiencies, improved sales tactics, and revenue growth. They may know that employee engagement and benefits are important, but they prefer to leave it to HR. This is a missed opportunity. High employee engagement is linked to many better business outcomes, including decreased turnover, increased employee ROI, and higher productivity, all of which end up benefiting the company's bottom line. And a good employee benefits plan is a crucial piece of employee engagement and satisfaction.

Unfortunately, CEOs and CFOs often do not realize the importance of their role in employee engagement. Studies consistently show that having top-level support for any company initiative is imperative to success. If the CEO and CFO visibly support a program, others throughout the company will too.

This is especially important when implementing a new solution, such as telehealth. Telehealth has the potential to be a game changer for a company's employee benefits plan. It can reduce health care costs for employers and employees, increase productivity, and reduce financial stress. But because it is so new, it needs an internal champion to ensure its success. CEOs and CFOs need to be a part of the process for choosing and promoting a telehealth solution. Only when the top executives have some ownership in the solution will telehealth's benefits be maximized.

Executives Need to Be Involved in the Decision Making

Employee benefit costs, particularly health care costs, have risen dramatically in recent years for both employers and employees. They are accounting for a larger and larger piece of total employee cost, second to payroll. But still, many CEOs and CFOs are not actively involved in choosing their employee benefits package. They may have certain numbers and targets they want to meet, but most rely heavily on the head of human resources and their employee benefits broker to effectively manage their benefits package. This process may have worked well in the past when benefits packages were more standard and traditional. But the workplace and health care landscape has changed dramatically in recent years. Employee loyalty is an issue, and medical costs are a challenge for many employees. Companies need new, innovative solutions that employees actually use and benefit from in order to increase retention and satisfaction. Sadly, HR and employee benefits brokers are not equipped to navigate this new environment.

Employee benefits brokers are typically seen as the industry experts. But they can only know and do so much. With ever-changing health care regulations and requirements, many already have their hands full with health insurance plans. They're not spending their free time learning about the newest ideas or innovations in employee benefits. As we discussed earlier in the book, brokers do not make that much money off these benefits. It is not worth their time to learn about them and then sell them to their clients, even if it's in their clients' best interests. This is especially true for smaller, regional brokers that many midsize companies use. If they are a company's main source of employee benefit ideas, there will be gaps in what is offered.

In HR, it's a similar story. HR departments are not known for having analytical and innovative mind-sets. They are *people* people. Their purpose is to help employees navigate the corporate systems and to help with administration. They are *not* there to innovate or analyze employee benefits. But creating a benefits package that fits the budget yet still attracts top level talent is a challenge. It requires a careful cost-benefit analysis that often involves qualitative and quantitative metrics. It does not fit with the HR skill set, which is why so many HR teams struggle to properly construct the right solution, let alone communicate effectively to get top-level executive buy-in. It's no surprise that most benefits packages are not meeting their goals.

Unfortunately, these two groups are exactly who CEOs and CFOs are relying on for their employee benefits package. It's become almost a habit for the top level of the company to just trust what HR and the brokers say and not spend any more time on it. But with the costs of benefits increasing faster than employee productivity, CEOs and CFOs must become more involved to ensure the continued success of their company and benefits package. They will be able to more creatively explore possible solutions, analyze the impact of different strategies, and choose what will work best in the short and long term for the company. Telehealth is one of those solutions that will appeal to many executives, especially those with self-funded or self-insured health insurance plans.

As costs have risen, more companies have switched to a self-funded health insurance model, and the trends indicate that more companies will continue to do so. For these companies, telehealth becomes an even more valuable benefit. At self-funded companies, the company is directly paying all of the health insurance claims from employee medical care. The actual health insurer is essentially the administrator of the plan. When it comes to telehealth, this means that every time an employee uses telehealth instead of a more expensive in-person visit, the employer pockets the difference. This directly affects the bottom line of an employer's health insurance costs. CEOs and CFOs need to recognize this and the power this benefit could have on their workforce.

Executives Need to Be Telehealth Champions

While being involved in the decision making is the first step for executives, their role should not end there. Too often they get caught up in financial targets and high-level company strategy.

They forget that they are not only the head of the company to outside investors and customers but to their employees as well. The CEO and executive team set the tone for the culture of the company. They have tremendous power to influence their employees, which is especially important for employee engagement initiatives. Without executive-level buy-in, many initiatives are sadly doomed to fail. New programs and solutions need an executive champion to communicate that it is important, and employees need to take notice.

Do you want employees to take the annual Voice of the Employee survey seriously? Make sure the CEO is asking people to take it, presenting on the results and next steps, and living the ideals. Do you want employees to use the new telehealth solution that the company just implemented? Have the CEO talk about it and promote it. When the CEO of a company gets involved in a program, the results are significantly greater than when the initiative only comes from HR. Visible CEO leadership inspires trust and confidence in a solution, which is critical when trying to get an entire employee population to change their health care habits. When CEOs get involved, engagement and utilization rates are measurably higher. And the benefits are tangible for a CEO or CFO. Their health care spending will go down. Employee absenteeism and unplanned time off will be reduced. Productivity and employee satisfaction will go up. This adds up to a better bottom line.

CEOs and CFOs need to take notice of the benefits that implementing and championing a telehealth solution can bring. This solution aligns with many high-level company goals around employee satisfaction *and* reducing costs to improve their profit margin. But to reap all of these benefits, they need to get involved. This includes sitting in on meetings with the provider, so they understand the solution and how it works. Then they need to visibly support the program. Depending on the company, this could mean a company-wide e-mail from the CEO himself, maybe including a personal use story. Or it could be announcing it at a quarterly all-company meeting. There are a lot of ways to easily show support without taking too much time. The small level of effort will amplify the success of the telehealth solution.

Working Directly with Telehealth Providers

This scenario happens all too often to me: I get in front of the CEO or CFO to present about telehealth and why it would be such a great benefit for them. They're engaged, they think it sounds great, but then at the end of the meeting, they want to go talk to their employee benefits broker about it. I get it. Executives are used to their broker handling all aspects of employee benefits. They are supposed to be experts in the field, and they should be able to tell the employer an unbiased opinion on it. However, in reality, what trying to work through your broker does is make the benefit more expensive, slow down the process, and overcomplicate it by adding another middleman.

Brokers are great for complex benefits. They negotiate with insurance companies on employers' behalf, which often results in lower rates for the employer than if they went directly to the provider. But brokers typically get paid a commission by the insurance providers as a percentage of total employer premium. So even though there is an additional cost baked into the employer's premiums, the broker's knowledge and relationships will still result in a better plan and a better deal for health insurance.

The same is not true for telehealth. It's a relatively straightforward solution. It's a per-employee-per-month fee that gives employees and their families access to the same benefit. There are not tons of plan design options and complex underwriting. So, there is no need for a broker to negotiate on the employer's behalf. Plain and simple, telehealth will be cheaper for employers if they work directly with the provider. Otherwise, the broker's cost will be included in the PEPMs.

Working through your broker also unnecessarily complicates and slows the process. Telehealth does not have to be implemented during annual enrollment. It can be started at any point throughout the year. In fact, we actually think that implementing the benefit off-cycle can be beneficial. There is less noise about other benefits, allowing more focus and attention to be on telehealth. So the sooner you can implement telehealth, the sooner employers and employees can start saving money. But working with a broker will add unnecessary steps and overcomplicate the entire process. Most are not well educated in telehealth. But they won't want to appear unknowledgeable to their clients. This means they will drag their feet at the beginning of the process as they try to learn about the industry, how providers differ, and how to evaluate different solutions. Once the process finally gets started, they are an unnecessary middleman that documents will have to go through, another level of approval to get, and another team to try and schedule meetings with.

Implementing telehealth should be easy and fast. But adding in the employee benefits broker will only slow it down.

With just a few due diligence steps to ensure the telehealth provider is good, employers can easily bypass employee benefits brokers to choose a telehealth provider themselves. It will save employers even more money and helps move the implementation process along quickly.

A Call to Action for CEOs and CFOs

Employee benefits and employer health care costs are a rising problem for CEOs and CFOs. Instead of depending on HR and an employee benefits broker to figure it out, executives need to take a more active role in choosing and championing new benefits, including telehealth. This solution has the potential to directly affect the employer's bottom line, all while providing a useful benefit to all employees. Instead of attempting to reduce costs by reducing benefits, telehealth can improve employee access to care and reduce employer costs at the same time. But CEOs and CFOs need to get engaged in the process in order to understand the impact this benefit can have on their company. Their support will make telehealth a success.

CHAPTER 10

Are All Telehealth Companies the Same?

When employers or brokers are considering a telehealth solution, many do not do their due diligence on evaluating competitors. After all, at first glance all of the solutions appear fairly similar. The patient signs up for the program, dials the phone number, and then speaks directly to a doctor. How many variations could there be? The broker and employer are already busy, and it is a low-cost (and therefore sometimes low priority) benefit. They decide to just choose the cheapest option or biggest player, if they even look at more than one solution. Unfortunately, when employers and brokers have this view, their telehealth results are often poor.

Despite offering a similar core service, there are key differences in the pricing, availability, and experience of various telehealth solutions. And these all affect an employer's utilization rate, which is the number-one success metric of telehealth. Understanding the differences between telehealth providers and how they affect utilization will allow employers and brokers to choose the best solution that will accomplish their goals of reducing costs and increasing access to care.

Fee per Use versus Zero Co-Pay

The biggest difference between various telehealth providers is their cost structure. The two most common are fee per use and zero co-pay. In a fee-per-use model, there is a co-pay every time that an individual has a virtual consultation. This can range from around thirty to sixty dollars per call. Some employers pay this fee for their employees, but that is not common. These solutions also have either a very low PEPM cost, one to two dollars, or no monthly cost. In a zero co-pay model, virtual consultations are free, but the PEPM is slightly higher to account for that, typically around three to ten dollars.

The problem with the fee-per-use model is that the employee co-pay discourages utilization. Having an up-front cost is a tough hurdle to overcome for all new services, let alone when it comes to health care. Think about all of the marketing for various services in the world. Many of them offer free trials or discounted rates for the first month or week. It is a well-documented psychological phenomenon that it is hard to get people to pay for a service that they have not used before. This problem is magnified in health care, where the service is personal as well as time sensitive. Not to mention that not every medical condition can be addressed by telehealth. Who wants to pay forty dollars to speak to a doctor, only to have the doctor tell you that you need to go to an urgent care (and likely pay an additional co-pay there)? This barrier is nearly impossible to overcome for employees, which is why these models almost always have very low utilization rates. The zero co-pay model, on the other hand, removes this barrier, and as a result shows much higher utilization.

Unfortunately, because of the higher up-front cost, many employers opt for the fee-per-use model over the zero co-pay solutions. Just like the trend in many other areas of employer-provided health insurance, it is another method of shifting cost onto employees. But with employees already stressed about medical costs, employers are missing a big opportunity. Zero co-pay telehealth reduces financial stress for employees and increases productivity by reducing sick time for doctor's visits. It is a meaningful benefit for employees, and it comes at very little incremental cost to the employer.

Limited versus Unlimited Consultations

Another difference between telehealth companies is whether or not they offer unlimited consultations. This is one of those small details that is often hidden in the fine print of a telehealth provider's offer. Clearly, unlimited consultations are preferable compared to a limited number of consultations.

By limiting consultations, the telehealth provider is essentially capping the amount of time and money savings employees *and* employers can reap by using telehealth. The telehealth provider may say that "it's rare an employee reaches these caps," trying to reassure the prospective client that it will not affect employees. If that is the case, employers should look carefully at that telehealth provider's utilization rates. Employers should want employees to use the solution. Otherwise what is the point of implementing it in the first place?

Often in this type of solution, the employee is not cut off after a certain number of visits. Instead, a surcharge is implemented for either the employer or employee after the limit has been reached. These charges often come as a nasty surprise. Employers and employees should not be penalized for using a solution they are already paying for. Brokers and employers need to read the fine print on telehealth solutions to check for overuse fees or consultation limits.

Employee Only versus Entire Family

Some telehealth providers have another sneaky way of limiting utilization—they only provide the solution to the covered employee, not the entire dependent family. While providing some telehealth may be better than nothing, employers are missing on savings by limiting the solution to only employees. In fact, since children are the most likely to get ill because of all the germs floating around at daycare and school, families with children are often the ones who most stand to benefit from a telehealth solution.

A recent survey by the University of Michigan uncovered some disappointing statistics: for parents with a child under six years old, a third of the parents reported missing work to care for a child. A quarter of the total parents had missed work three or more times in the past year to care for a child. And eight percent reported that the emergency room was more convenient than their primary-care options. That is a lot of time and money wasted on what are typically normal illnesses, such as the cold, flu, or pinkeye.

One of the best ways to reduce parental PTO for a sick child is by early diagnosis and treatment. But because of the cost and time to access medical care, many parents delay seeking treatment. They want to see if their child gets better on their own, maybe after they sleep. But starting an antibiotic early can often keep the child healthier and keep them in school or daycare, eliminating the need for the parent to take a sick day.

Providing the entire family with telehealth does, naturally, raise the cost of the solution. But the benefits can be exponential for those families with children. It is the best way for employers to see increased productivity and less stress from their employees.

Claims versus No Claims

A hidden catch of telehealth solutions is whether or not the virtual consultation generates a claim. This is a problem with many solutions that are embedded in employer health insurance plans. Because the consultation occurs through the health insurance company, the health insurer wants the call to generate a claim, just as any other in-person visit would. On the other hand, independent telehealth solutions often work entirely separately of health insurance and do not generate a claim. Those solutions are preferable, because generating a claim for each consultation is not as effective at reducing costs for employees or employers.

From an employee perspective, the virtual consultation ends up being almost as expensive as an in-person visit. There is likely a co-pay, and then the employee will get a medical bill from his or her health insurer in the mail weeks later. This is a tough pill to swallow, especially given how new the service is to most employees. They are already skeptical. If the cost savings are not substantial, it will be hard to convince them to use the solution. Utilization will take a hit.

From an employer perspective, it also ends up being almost as expensive, especially if the company is self-funded since they are paying the health insurer's share of the claim. An additional issue for employers is that by not reducing the total number of claims, they are missing an opportunity to negotiate a lower renewal price for their health insurance. Every year, an employer's incumbent health insurer reviews their claim history to determine what the next year's employer and employee premiums should be. If a lot of employees got sick that year and generated claims, premiums will go up. But if employers implement a solution that actually *reduces* the number of claims, such as independent telehealth, employers can better negotiate for a lower premium.

Most telehealth implemented in the market today is embedded in health insurance. But employees and employers are losing out on one of the best potential benefits of telehealth when these solutions are chosen. Independent telehealth solutions that do not generate a claim are the most effective at reducing costs in the short and long term.

No Accountability versus Accountability

Who is accountable for the success of the telehealth solution? I've said it before, but it is worth repeating. Unless someone is held responsible for the success of a telehealth program, it will likely fail. And the best group for that accountability is the telehealth provider itself. It is the only way that employers and brokers can be confident that the provider will do whatever it can to ensure the solution's success.

When a telehealth provider is not held responsible for their solution's performance, they typically engage as little as possible with the employer or employees once the solution has been sold. They do not help with implementation. They do not help with a communication strategy. Instead, they let the employer dump the entire responsibility onto the HR department, where it almost inevitably fails. The HR department is not a marketing department, and they are not telehealth experts. They do not know how to drive utilization and results, if they even try to.

With a telehealth provider that does hold itself accountable for results, the experience is much different. They will be heavily involved in implementation to ensure employee participation and sign up. Throughout the year, they will communicate with employees to drive utilization and to keep the solution top-of-mind. Their communication pieces will be timely, relevant, and will educate the employees on how, why, and when to use telehealth. The communication strategy will be specifically developed to drive results. Even better is a telehealth provider that holds itself *financially* accountable to their clients' results. Their commitment to outcomes becomes apparent in implementations, communication strategies, and user experience.

Good versus Bad User Experience

A critical component to a successful telehealth solution is the user experience. While in theory the telehealth services are the same—there is a phone number you call—the actual user experience can be quite different in reality.

With a bad user experience, employees may find it difficult or time consuming to sign up or register for the solution. There may even be a waiting period after signup before they can have a consultation. Wait times are often long and the quality of the visits, poor. It is a frustrating experience that does not turn employees into repeat telehealth patients.

One of the tricks that some providers use is a custom portal or user experience. They will design a web interface that is branded for a specific company. It may seem like special treatment, but the only thing special is the portal branding. Once the employee calls, he or she is in the same waiting room as everyone else. It is not an employer-specific solution.

What employers should look for instead is a web portal that is easy to use and consumer friendly. Employees should be able to sign up and have a consultation on the same day. The sign up should be fast and easy. Wait times should be short, and the company should have various quality assurance methods. A combination of rating systems and consultation reviews works well. The doctors should also be trained specifically in how to conduct virtual consultations. They should have the latest trainings and resources available in order to practice the best telehealth they can.

At the end of the day, a great user experience is what brings a customer back. Getting an employee to sign up and try telehealth is the first, and often greatest, challenge. But employers, brokers, and providers need to look beyond initial sign up. User experience and satisfaction needs to be considered to ensure that the solution is meeting patient needs. Only then will telehealth be able to transform how an employee population accesses health care.

It All Comes Down to Utilization

The differences in telehealth providers may seem small, but each one determines how effective a solution can be. All of these factors influence the utilization rate. Without high utilization, telehealth becomes just another wasted service that employers and employees are paying for.

Sadly, many employers and brokers are not knowledgeable enough about telehealth to detect these differences. Many simply choose the lowest-cost provider. But with that comes additional employee fees, limited consultations for employees only, more claims, no support, and a bad user experience. Instead, employers should opt for the telehealth solution that will deliver a superior product with better and guaranteed results.

CHAPTER 11

OBJECTIONS TO TELEHEALTH

Almost everyone agrees that telehealth is the way of the future. And while most of the obstacles to telehealth's success have been created by bad solutions and lack of employer education, there are also fears about telehealth that have stood in its way. But every new technology has faced criticism and skepticism. These objections are mainly based on fear and resistance to change. Without knowing the full story of telehealth and virtual consultations, like how to use it and the way it works, some have dismissed the solution as a whole. And while telehealth is by no means a replacement for all medical care or all general practitioner visits, when used correctly, it is a life-changing solution for millions of people who struggle with the time and money traditional health care takes. So, let's look at these objections and debunk them.

The Physician-Patient Relationship

One of the biggest criticisms of telehealth is that it erodes the physician-patient relationship. In an ideal world, your general practitioner or pediatrician will have been with you or your children for years. They know and remember your medical history and can ask better questions because of it. They know your family medical history, and maybe you even run into them at the grocery store. They may know you so well that they're able to detect changes in you that even you haven't noticed yet.

This sounds great, but it's not the case for the majority of people. Convenience and ease of access trumps the traditional relationship. There are large percentages of the population, 28 percent of men and 17 percent of all women, that don't even have a primary care physician. It's even worse among millennials: 28 percent don't have a primary-care doctor, and an *additional* 40 percent don't have a relationship with their primary care physician. So even if someone has an established primary care doctor, he or she may not see the doctor often enough to develop a relationship. The story of the doctor who knows you is less and less common. One of the main causes of this decline is the shortage of primary care physicians. The current average wait time to see a general practitioner is nineteen days. And that number is increasing. When you're sick, you can't wait nineteen days to see a doctor. And then you only end up spending maybe fifteen minutes with the doctor anyway because he or she is so tightly booked. Instead, you'll find the care you need somewhere else.

That's why people are using walk-in clinics, urgent cares, and ERs for many nonurgent medical needs. Even if your physician is part of a physician's group that may have a same-day center, you likely won't be seeing your regular doctor. The truth is, for most people, there is no real physician-patient relationship to erode.

People will get care wherever is most convenient. Telehealth is rarely displacing a visit to a primary care doctor; it is more often replacing unnecessary and expensive urgent care and ER visits.

Continuity of Care

Related to the physician-patient relationship is a worry about the continuity of care when using telehealth. It's helpful to have a physician who knows you and your medical history, especially if you have interrelated health issues. If an illness doesn't get better even after a recommended treatment or you end up with a recurring illness, there is no doubt that having gone to only one doctor throughout would be helpful. But, same as before, this scenario is rarely happening. Even if you are one of those unlucky people who doesn't respond to treatment or has a pesky ear infection that always seems to be coming back, it's unlikely that you'd be going to the same doctor every time anyway. Plus, with some solutions, you have the option to send your primary care office a record of your virtual visit, including the diagnosis and recommended treatment. So, if you do end up needing to go to your primary care office, your doctor will already have the information from your previous consultation.

In the broader scope, telehealth is all about using communication to enhance health care. One of the problems facing the medical industry today is a lack of communication. Patients feel that their care is siloed; it doesn't appear that specialists and primary care doctors are communicating. Every time you go to an office visit, you have to fill out piles of paperwork answering the same questions over and over. And then the nurse and doctor will go over some of those questions *again*. Information from visits to urgent cares, ERs, and walk-in clinics aren't sent to the patient or their regular doctor. Patients often skip check-ins and have trouble with medication adherence, but it's too costly and time consuming to go to their doctor as regularly as they should. Increased use of communication technology in health care could help with all of these issues. Patients and doctors should be able to communicate more easily. And doctors and specialists need to be able to communicate effectively on a patient's health and treatments. Virtual consultations are a step in the right direction for facilitating increased communication between patients and health care professionals.

Quality of Care

Other critics worry about the quality of care available via telehealth, even though studies have consistently shown that the quality of health care services rendered via telehealth are as good as in-person visits. But still, without being able to see someone in person and feel their throat or inspect their ears, some people feel that the diagnoses and treatment recommendations cannot be satisfactory. However, this just isn't the case. Telehealth can adequately and appropriately diagnose and treat many common ailments. The symptoms are so telling and consistent that inspecting a patient in person isn't necessary. High-quality videoconferencing also makes visual inspection of a patient possible. Studies have shown that 65 percent of children's illnesses could be treated via telehealth and 38 percent of older adults' hospital visits could be replaced with telehealth. Additionally, over 70 percent of total urgent care and ER visits could be redirected to virtual consultations.[15]

Many physicians see the same cases over and over again. When it's flu season, doctors see flu patients every day. They'll recognize it and its symptoms even in a videoconference. Plus, how many times have you known ahead of time what you have? If you've had pinkeye once, you can recognize it in yourself or your children. You don't need to spend a lot of time and money for an in-person doctor to tell you what you already know! And for peace of mind, if the doctor is unsure, he will simply recommend visiting an in-person physician. Since telehealth visits only take a few minutes, you won't have lost much by trying a virtual visit first. It could save hours of your time.

To ensure high-quality care, you should look for a telehealth provider that cares about quality and has high patient satisfaction. You should also look for a telehealth solution that provides telehealth specific training to all physicians, so they are well-equipped to practice virtual medicine. All physicians must be licensed in the state they practice in and be US board certified. A company that also provides patient surveys and reviews selected consultations should be able to ensure that that consultations are meeting expectations. You can ask for a company's satisfaction and recommendation numbers to see how the end users rate their experience.

An added bonus is that by increasing the appropriate use of telehealth, the quality of care at in-person sites could actually improve. Right now, too many doctors are facing burnout. Urgent cares and ERs are distracted by the nonemergency cases that come seeking treatment. If unnecessary visits could be replaced by telehealth, doctors and nurses would have more time to focus on patients with conditions that really need their attention. This could increase physician engagement and reduce medical errors. In short, quality of care would increase.

Most illnesses simply don't need a physician to be physically with the patient to diagnose and recommend treatment. The quality of care in a virtual consultation is just as good in these circumstances as an in-person visit. And if patients switched to virtual consultations for these cases, quality of care at other sites of care could actually improve. It's a win-win situation for people's medical care.

Information Security
In the age of stolen identities and mass data-breach scares, many people are, understandably, worried about the security of their information when using telehealth. Speaking on the phone or using a videoconference to convey private and personal information seems risky. But telehealth companies have high-end security technology to keep your information safe.

For all healthcare information, companies must comply with the HIPAA Privacy Rule, which establishes a baseline level of protection. Because of the sensitivity of personal health data, telehealth companies should be HIPAA-compliant and take patient security seriously. Other states and local areas have even higher security standards. No matter where you live, your telehealth solution should meet the required security levels and be able to share information with your primary care while following all applicable laws. Even still, people do need to be educated about where and when you use telehealth. Sitting on the public Wi-Fi network in a crowded Starbucks while sharing your personal health data probably isn't a good decision. But the systems and portals themselves are safe and secure to use. Most of your health information is already online, either through your health insurance company or your doctor's office websites. The best way to protect yourself isn't to try and avoid having your data online—it's a lost cause for most of us—but to monitor your information closely, use good password strategies, and to use secure networks.

There Are No Real Concerns

When used appropriately, there are no real concerns about telehealth. Any fears are mostly rooted in fear of change and a lack of knowledge. It is a cost-effective, time-saving solution that will help millions of people get the care they need. It won't, and shouldn't, replace all in-person visits. It's a supplement that takes advantage of the great improvements in telecommunication technology and applies them to health care.

The current model is outdated and inconvenient for treating many of the common ailments that people seek medical care for. Technology and life has changed, and the way we access medical care needs to catch up. The reality is that most of us no longer have that family doctor that was easily accessible, knew all of our health conditions (and our mother's!), and who we went to for all of our medical needs. Our current care is already fragmented between walk-in clinics, urgent cares, specialists, and more. Virtual consultations will not change the dynamic we have with our primary cares. But it will enable people to easily get the medical attention they need. And unlike other sites of care, we'll even send the information to your primary care office so that your doctor is always in the loop.

CHAPTER 12

Telehealth FAQs

Even though the concept of virtual consultations for telehealth may be clear, many people still have questions about the details. Here are some of the most common questions about using telehealth. If you have questions that are not answered here or that are about a specific telehealth provider, you should first check their website and then reach out directly to the company with any further questions.

Who Are the Doctors?

US law requires that a doctor be licensed in the state he or she is practicing in. It does not matter whether the visit is virtual or in-person—the same laws apply. This means that all telehealth doctors are US board certified and licensed in the state in which the patient lives. The same should be true of all reputable telehealth companies. When you call in, you will only be connected with a doctor licensed in your state.

The doctors are available twenty-four hours a day, seven days a week, 365 days a year. Some providers allow you to schedule your virtual consultation in advance. You may even be able to browse the doctor profiles and select an appointment time and a practitioner of your choice. When making an unscheduled call, you will be placed with the first available doctor licensed in your state. Generally, any unscheduled consultation does *not* allow you to choose a specific doctor. This decreases overall average wait times and increases the efficiency of the solutions. Average wait times vary by provider, but it is typically less than fifteen minutes for an unscheduled call.

Some telehealth providers have expanded their services to include other medical specialties besides primary care. Some even offer access to board certified pharmacists, dentists, optometrists, dietitians, and sports medicine, alternative medicine, and mental health professionals. These specialists are also available 24/7/365 and do not require a patient to schedule in advance, but that is not true for all telehealth providers. Other telehealth providers may have some of these specialists available but only if scheduled in advance.

The doctors are the core of providing a valuable service to patients, so choose a company that takes care in selecting and evaluating the doctors in their network. The doctors should have access to the latest trainings on conducting virtual consultations. Many solutions also have a rating and review system for quality control and continuous improvement. Periodically reviewing entire recordings of virtual consultations is another best practice for a telehealth provider to deliver

. . .

When Should I Use Telehealth?

Telehealth *is not* for medical emergencies. If you suspect a medical emergency, always call 911 immediately.

Telehealth *is* for nonemergent medical issues, especially common illnesses and conditions. Telehealth doctors are all able to treat a wide range of patients and conditions. The most common conditions we treat are acne, allergies, constipations, cough, diarrhea, ear problems, fever, flu, headache, insect bite, nausea/vomiting, pinkeye, rash, respiratory problems, sore throats, urinary problems/UTIs, vaginitis, and more. By using telehealth for these common conditions instead of a primary care physician, urgent care, walk-in clinic, or emergency room, patients can save valuable time and money. Most primary care doctors see these conditions every day. In most cases, they are easily recognizable based on symptom descriptions and video inspection. Treatment plans are straightforward, and if a prescription is necessary, the telehealth doctor can send it electronically to the patient's pharmacy of choice. If the doctor is unsure or thinks that further physical examination is necessary, the patient will be directed to see a doctor in person. This is one of the main reasons to choose a solution that does not charge per virtual consultation. Not all conditions will be able to be treated virtually (although our current issue resolution rate is 94 percent), so this avoids a patient being double charged for the same condition.

Telehealth is also great to use when traveling, when finding a local site of care is even more complicated. The telehealth doctors can diagnose patients when they're on the road, so they can get the treatment they need right away instead of waiting until they are home. This means they get better faster and without wasting a lot of time trying to find care in an unfamiliar city.

Is the Quality of Care as Good?

While using a phone call or videoconference to diagnose and treat a condition may seem odd at first, the quality of telehealth care has been documented to be as effective as in-person care. Most of the conditions are extremely common, and doctors see thousands of patients with the same thing every year. However, as with any health care visit, whether in person or virtual, patients should come prepared with questions, list all current medications and allergies, and listen carefully to treatment instructions. Additionally, technological improvements and new innovations will continue to improve the potential and quality of telehealth consultations. And if a patient is deciding between telehealth and no care at all, telehealth has a clear positive effect on health outcomes.

The American Telemedicine Association has also created a set of standards, guidelines, and best practices for telehealth solutions. These are guided by their years of research and expertise. This ensures that providers are using telehealth effectively and responsibly.

How Do I Access a Telehealth Doctor?

Most telehealth solutions are simple to access and are designed both for patients who are tech savvy and those who are not. Most solutions have a website and/or app as well as a telephone number. The website or app enables videoconferencing, which can help with diagnosing more conditions. But for less tech-savvy individuals, the telephone number is also available.

Depending on the solution, you may or may not need to provide health insurance information. With standalone solutions, it is not normally required, which makes sign up quick and easy. Patients can be talking to a doctor within minutes of activating their account. There is also the ability to fill out a medical history profile, which will enable the doctor to be better prepared for the appointment.

Telehealth solutions can be accessed on most mobile and tablet devices with an Internet connection. Some providers will list specific system requirements if using videoconferencing. To get the best results from a phone call or videoconference, you need the same thing you need for any other phone call or Skype visit. You need a strong Internet connection or good cell-phone service, a high-quality webcam, a working microphone, and adequate speakers. Some solutions have equipment tests that you can run on your computer before conducting a visit, so you can ensure you have the technology capabilities and correct set-up.

How Do Prescriptions Work?

Telehealth doctors are able to write prescriptions for nonnarcotic medications via a virtual consultation. Drugs that cannot be prescribed are those that are considered controlled substances by the DEA and/or may be harmful because of the potential for abuse. This includes, for example, antidepressant drugs such as Prozac and Zoloft as well as antianxiety medications such as

Xanax. The most commonly prescribed medications via telehealth are antibiotics, prescription-strength rash creams, and eye or ear drops.

If the telehealth doctor deems a prescription necessary for treatment, the prescription can be sent electronically to the patient's pharmacy. If a patient's preferred pharmacy is not available, a traditional prescription can be filled by the doctor and then faxed to that pharmacy. All prescriptions are fully compliant and include all required information.

How Much Does Telehealth Cost?

As discussed extensively throughout the book, different telehealth solutions have different cost structures. With standalone solutions, there is a flat monthly cost that covers unlimited telehealth consultations. This cost may be covered by an employer, which makes the service completely free for the employee. Some solutions are also directly available to the consumer, so an individual may sign up through our website or phone number.

With the direct-to-consumer offerings, there are individual and family plans. Both include virtual consultations with doctors and specialists, but some solutions have limits and others do not. Payment is typically not needed until an individual actually schedules a consultation. If scheduling an appointment in advance, some solutions even allow for refunds, granted you cancel at least twenty-four hours before the scheduled appointment. Most solutions accept most all major credit cards.

Not all solutions are as straightforward with their pricing. Some solutions may have an individual co-pay for each consultation in addition to the flat monthly cost. Other solutions may generate an insurance claim, and the patient will be billed through their health insurance provider similarly to an in-person visit. Before choosing a solution for you or your family, make sure you understand every cost associated with using the solution.

What Limits Are There?

To maximize the benefits of telehealth, there should be no limits on usage. Unfortunately, not every telehealth provider feels that way. Some provide unlimited virtual consultations with one monthly fee, either individual or family. While others charge for each consultation creating a barrier to utilization. Patients should not need to worry about wasting one of their calls if they are unsure whether they need to see a doctor. Families with multiple kids do not have to worry about running out of visits when one child gets sick, since we all know that means the whole family will probably end up sick! Other telehealth providers often try to limit the virtual consultations. They may place an individual call limit on a monthly or annual basis. Or they may charge an excess utilization fee for individuals or employers if the solution is being used too frequently. This obviously limits the potential benefit of the solution for both individuals and employers and is an important feature to examine when selecting a solution.

Is Telehealth Private and Secure?

All telehealth solutions have to comply with applicable HIPAA laws that establish minimum security guidelines for private health information. While there can be no guarantees for any private information, online or not, these laws were put in place by the government to protect individuals' personal health information. So, these telehealth solutions are as secure as any other hospital's or insurer's online portals. That being said, patients should take care with where they conduct their telehealth sessions. Patients should use a personal, secure wireless Internet connection, not the local library or coffee shop.

CHAPTER 13

How to Choose Between an On-Site Clinic and Telehealth

As health care costs for employers and employees have continued to grow, HR has struggled to find effective cost-containment solutions. While many employers have simply tried to shift costs and responsibility to employees, other employers have been looking for innovative solutions. In addition to telehealth, one of the more popular ideas in recent years has been the implementation of on-site clinics.

These clinics bring primary care to the workplace, making care more convenient and economical for employees. These clinics seem attractive to many employers, especially large employers with the majority of their employees at one location. But while on-site clinics certainly have benefits, they also have many drawbacks and shortcomings, especially when compared to a telehealth solution. Employers need to carefully consider each solution to determine which is the best for their company and their employees.

Availability

The promise of an on-site clinic is easy access to care during the workday. Instead of driving thirty minutes each way to a doctor, employees can simply walk to the clinic in their building. Unfortunately, due to limited hours and availability, on-site clinics fall short of telehealth for making health care more convenient.

On-site clinics, due to a limited patient population, usually have a very small staff and limited hours of operation. If the schedule is full or a patient needs care on a day that the clinic is not open, the patient is out of luck. Employees will either have to wait for care or use another site of care, which diminishes the benefit of the on-site clinic. Similarly, if a patient needs care in the evening, on a weekend, during vacation, or during a holiday, the clinic will be no help. The employee will have to spend valuable time and money visiting an emergency room or urgent care.

Balancing supply and demand for on-site clinics is a constant challenge. On the one hand, if the clinic is not 100 percent utilized during open hours, the employer is still paying wages and utility costs for the hours the clinic is open, whether or not an employee is receiving care. But on the other hand, if a clinic is always busy, employees will struggle to schedule last-minute appointments. The whole point of an on-site clinic is to make care more convenient, and a clinic that has long wait times misses the mark.

The value of on-site clinic is also limited to employees who are in the office. What about patients who are too sick to be in the office? No one wants to potentially run into an executive or a boss when they are not feeling well. So employees that do not want to visit the office to get care cannot take advantage of this benefit. They are stuck with the traditional options of urgent cares, walk-in clinics, and emergency rooms. Spouses and children also do not benefit much from on-site clinics. While technically many of these clinics allow family members, spouses and children may not want to get medical care at an office. Most people do not want to bring a sick, fussy child to a parent's place of work. Or a spouse may not want his or her spouse's coworkers seeing him or her sick. For many family members, it would be uncomfortable to use the on-site clinic. Even for those families who do not mind visiting the office for care, the clinic is not actually that convenient for them. There is still a drive into the office, which may be far away, even if the wait times are shorter than other sites of care. Overall, families and employees who truly are not feeling well likely will not find the office a convenient spot for medical care.

A last limitation on availability of on-site clinics is for remote employees. Whether an employee works entirely at home, works in a satellite office, or simply travels a lot for work, that employee will not benefit from the on-site clinic. As working remotely and working from home grow more popular, the value of on-site clinics diminishes by excluding a portion of employees.

On the other hand, telehealth is available every hour of every day of the year. It is accessible for every employee and every covered family member, no matter where they are located. Wait times are short, and most consultations do not take long, either.

On-site clinics are certainly convenient and can reduce employees' health care costs when they can actually be used. Unfortunately, there are so many limitations to when and who can use them, that the potential benefit is limited. Telehealth, on the other hand, has fewer limitations and thus more potential to benefit your employees by reducing the time and cost of care.

Available Services

In some respects, on-site clinics have more thorough primary care services than telehealth. Many of the clinics function as full-service primary care offices. They can do routine visits, such as biometric testing and annual physicals. They can also treat a broader range of acute illnesses and conditions, because the doctors and nurses can feel for symptoms, check the ears and throat, listen to breathing, and more. The clinics may also be able to provide vaccinations and lab tests. And for patients with chronic conditions, they offer convenient access to the same physician to improve continuity of care.

Telehealth, however, is not designed to entirely replace a person's primary care. It cannot be used for annual physicals, biometric testing, or vaccinations. It is best used for acute illnesses and conditions. But with telehealth, the doctors are limited by what symptoms they can physically see and what the patient can describe. This may seem like a significant drawback, but in reality, the majority of conditions that primary care doctors see can be effectively diagnosed and treated remotely. These conditions are common and routine, and the doctors recognize them easily. Seeing an in-person physician is simply not necessary the majority of the time. So yes, telehealth has some limitations that an on-site clinic does not, but these instances are a very small percentage of overall primary care visits.

But that is not the entire story on services. In fact, some telehealth solutions offer a much broader range of services than on-site clinics by providing access to specialists. Members can now speak to psychiatrists, counselors, nutritionists, physical therapists, dentists, optometrists, and more using the same telehealth service. This access dramatically increases the scope of how telehealth can affect and improve employee's access to medical care. There are very few on-site clinics that can deliver this range of specialty services.

Additionally, technology and innovation in telehealth improve every day. The number and type of conditions that can be diagnosed and treated remotely continues to grow. A solution that an employer implements today can give employees access to a broad array of medical help and care, as well as the promise of even better and more comprehensive service in the future.

Implementation

Perhaps the biggest drawback of an on-site clinic compared to a telehealth solution is the up-front implementation cost, both in time and capital. The up-front costs are immense, because a physical space needs to be built and equipped. When you truly start to think about what all is involved in developing an on-site clinic, the costs and complications add up quickly.

To start with, an employer needs to allocate or develop new space within their building for the clinic. The clinic needs three rooms, at the minimum: a waiting room, an administrative room, and an exam room. Office space is not inexpensive, and the opportunity cost of using this space for a clinic as opposed to offices needs to be built into the calculations. Plus, the space needs to be built specifically for medical needs, which require a different architecture, engineering, and construction than a typical office building. Once a space has been built, it needs to be filled with medical supplies and expensive medical equipment. After the clinic has been built and equipped, staff, including expensive physicians, need to be hired. This means there are ongoing costs including wages, utilities, and supply costs. The costs are high, which means that the benefits will not outweigh the initial capital costs for years. All of this adds up to a very expensive benefit, not to mention the time involved.

Planning, building, executing, and managing a project of this magnitude requires a lot of hours and manpower. Unless an employer hires a consultant to oversee the project, which is an added expense, that time is taken away from other important internal projects. Building an on-site clinic takes months. If you factor in the entire process, from discussions to approvals and finding capital to the actual opening, the time horizon becomes even longer.

Telehealth, however, is inexpensive and easy to implement. It is a simple per-employee-per-month fee, with no up-front capital expenditure needed. The solution can be implemented at any time of year, and implementation is fast and easy. Savings start as soon as the first employee uses telehealth instead of an urgent care, which could be just a few weeks after making the decision to go ahead with telehealth. And depending on the telehealth provider an employer chooses, the employer and HR may have very little to do for the implementation. The best telehealth providers do the heavy lifting for implementations and employee engagement campaigns, allowing HR to focus on their other priorities.

Savings and Value

When employers are looking to implement a new, innovative employee benefit, the number-one thing they are normally looking for is return on investment. The savings generated by the investment need to be worth the money.

On-site clinics clearly have value. An individual visit at the clinic is cheaper than care provided by another physician. It reduces time away from work. Over time, it can even help improve overall employee health. But because of the extensive up-front cost, both in capital and time invested, seeing a positive ROI on a clinic can take a long time. Also, calculating the ROI is not straightforward. Most companies that help employers develop on-site clinics have complicated ROI calculations that include savings generated by reduced absenteeism and improved employee health. While these are important features of any employee benefit, these "savings" are mostly guesswork, not true bottom-line savings.

With telehealth, employers can see a positive ROI in the *first year*. Every time an employee uses telehealth instead of an in-person visit, the employer saves money. With a highly utilized solution, the savings add up quickly, especially since telehealth is always available. Because telehealth can be used by any family member, anywhere, at any time of the day, a larger percentage of visits can be diverted to the lower cost site of care than with an on-site clinic. And calculating the ROI is straightforward—it's the cost of avoided in-person visits minus the cost of telehealth. But that does not mean that the other "soft" benefits are not there. Just like an on-site clinic, telehealth will reduce absenteeism due to medical visits and improve overall employee health. It also reduces the financial and emotional stress of medical care for many employees. But unlike on-site clinics, telehealth does not have to resort to quantifying these soft benefits to try and justify its ROI. The bottom-line financials for telehealth speak for themselves.

Telehealth Comes Out Ahead

While on-site clinics can provide value for the right company and the right employee demographic, telehealth is an equally valuable solution, at a much lower price point. So, companies that are looking for ways to improve access for employees while reducing health care costs should first look to telehealth instead. Telehealth has the ability to reduce costs and show a positive return on investment in the first year, not to mention the value it brings to employees and their families. It is fast and inexpensive to implement, making it easier to gain internal buy-in and to move quickly on an innovative solution. Companies can improve their employees' benefits in just weeks, not months. Telehealth is an easy choice for companies that are looking to improve their health care costs and benefits.

CHAPTER 14

How Telehealth Is Transforming Health Care

Health care in America needs to be fixed. No one doubts that. The government can try to fix it through various regulations, laws, and mandates, but none of these will actually fix any of the root problems. While health insurance companies are not blameless, they are not the only reason that our current system is not working for everyone. Our current system is outdated and is not using technological developments to its full advantage. If the medical industry embraced technology and started using telehealth, the health care of the future could look very different than it does today. That is how powerful telehealth could be.

Different Site of Care Needs

Today, there's a shortage of primary care doctors, ERs are overcrowded, and rural populations struggle to get access to specialists. Increased use of telehealth could change the current problems and shortcomings of today's sites of care.

Emergency rooms are struggling with overcrowding. Part of the problem is the high number of patients that do not actually need emergency room treatment. In fact, over 12 percent of ER cases are nonemergency. This is caused by many things. Some patients have problems in the middle of the night, and the emergency room is the only place open. The problem may not actually be an emergency, but the patient is operating by the "better safe than sorry" mantra. Other patients simply may not be educated on their other health care options. If the emergency room is close by, they may just go there first. Then there are the patients that cannot afford care. ERs cannot turn patients away, so even patients who know they will not be able to afford treatment may end up at the ER. Because of this, many hospitals are struggling with appropriate staffing and maintaining profitability in the ERs. Nurses and doctors are overworked, but because of the lower profitability of patients who are unable to pay or have lower-cost medical problems, hospitals cannot increase the staffing. But with telehealth, these patients will be able to quickly access the care they need without overburdening ERs. And if it becomes widespread enough, it will be a cost-effective solution for many patients who currently struggle to pay medical bills. Over time, this will positively affect the effectiveness and needs of ERs.

Primary care practices are also facing difficulties because of the shortage of primary care physicians. Average wait times are weeks long for an appointment in cities, but rural doctors occasionally struggle with *enough* volume. But using telehealth will spread the patient needs and distribute the workload more evenly. Primary care doctors in smaller areas will be able to supplement their local practice with telehealth consultations in other parts of the state. Primary care practices in crowded cities will benefit from these common conditions being treated virtually, freeing up their time to see the patients that need in-person care sooner.

Another site-of-care challenge in the current health care environment is access to specialists. Currently, in rural areas, patients do not have convenient access to the specialists they need. A doctor's appointment is already time consuming and inconvenient enough—just imagine if you had to see a specialist who was two hours away! Telehealth can help address this issue in two major ways. First, at-home technology may advance enough for certain specialties to be conducted completely remotely, from the patient's home. Some of these are already happening, such as dietitians, mental health specialists, and even dermatologists. There are remote dermatology services that allow patients to upload pictures of a skin concern for a dermatologist to discuss with them and diagnose. With advances in technology and more at-home tools, these capabilities will only increase. Take, for example, a product called Oto. It connects to a smartphone camera and has a connected app that directs the user on how to take photos of the inner ear to send to a doctor. For parents with small children who frequently get ear infections, this can save a lot of time and money instead of going to the doctor. The second way telehealth improves access to specialists is by connecting a primary care facility or hospital to a specialist. In the above example, not every parent will have access to a smartphone or the Oto. But a primary care facility, walk-in clinic, or even a school nurse could. These images could be sent to a primary care doctor or even an ENT. This will greatly improve access to care for even more complicated and urgent concerns than can be treated at home.

Over time, these changes will affect specialists' practices and where they are located. For example, if 20 percent of dermatology visits could be completed virtually, there would likely be fewer dermatology offices, but a virtual dermatology center may pop up instead. There may be sophisticated algorithms that complete an initial diagnosis of a skin condition based on the pictures, which then determines which specialist it gets sent to. These dermatologists could all collaborate and learn from each other by being in a centralized location. In the current environment, there may be only one specialist in a twenty-five-mile radius. This limits his or her continuing education, professional discussions, or even second opinions. But a centralized, virtual group would lower overhead costs and foster communication between the specialists.

A great example of this already happening is in the ICU. Some hospitals have started implementing telehealth in their Intensive Care Units (ICU). These solutions allow vital signs and physiological status of ICU patients to be monitored continuously (and remotely) to identify recommended actions sooner. It's a combination of algorithms with doctors overseeing the programs to recommend specific actions. These programs have shown decreases in average length of stay and higher survival rates, because they allow fewer doctors to monitor more patients effectively. They are also in a centralized location where they can ask another doctor for an opinion and learn from each other. These types of remote monitoring facilities will change how staffing and management of current facilities are operated.

Increased Competition

Telehealth is increasing competition in health care, in more than just one way. Not only does it increase the health care options for patients, but it also will serve as an important differentiator for in-person providers.

Telehealth companies that provide virtual consultations are a new option for patients. That puts them in direct competition with hospitals, ERs, urgent cares, primary care offices, and walk-in clinics. While diverting visits from these expensive sites of care to telehealth will be good for the entire system, these facilities will still have to grapple with the financial impact of declining case volume. For example, diverting nonemergency cases away from the ER will help to give overworked nurses and doctors more time and better care to those that truly need emergency care. But many ERs are already struggling financially because so many ER patients to do not have enough money to pay their bills or they are Medicare patients, which means the reimbursements are lower. Reducing case volume may affect an ER's finances, and hospitals may have to rethink their ER strategy.

To address this, many large hospital systems are implementing their own telehealth solutions. Hospitals hope that by having their own platform and service, patients that typically come to their hospital or their hospital system will use their telehealth solution instead of a competitor's. These hospital-specific solutions may have another impact—it could increase their overall reach. Some of these solutions require an in-person visit first to establish the patient as a patient of that hospital system. But if they do not, there is nothing stopping someone from elsewhere in the state using that hospital's telehealth solution. If a hospital has a high reputation in a specific area, remote patients may want to use their telehealth solution to speak to experts in the field, instead of their local hospital. This could magnify the disparities between hospital systems over time, because patients will be able to choose the best care, not simply the closest care.

This leads into the second way telehealth will increase competition by becoming a differentiator for in-person providers. Currently, there often appear to be very few differentiators between physician groups. Many hospitals have strong (or weak) reputations. But primary care offices, dermatologists, or OB/GYN offices, for example, do not. For consumers, it was often a blind guess as to which doctor's office was better. The best a patient could hope for was a recommendation from a trusted friend or family member. Patients may have shopped around for a doctor they liked, but that was about it. Online reviews were a first step in providing patients with a guide for choosing the best care. But any differentiators in cost, outcome, wait times, and more are still hard to come by. There are websites out there that try to help, but most are not easy to use. With telehealth, a good telehealth solution will become an important differentiator for these sites of care.

Already, some primary care physicians are part of a group that has a same-day service center. They use this service as a way to stand out among other primary care offices. If your primary care doctor is unavailable when you need a same-day appointment, there are other primary care doctors in the same group that will be able to see you that same day. It is the same phone number, the same website, and the same cost—just a different doctor. This level of access is a powerful motivator for patients to use this group. Telehealth solutions will build on this. Doctors, physician groups, outpatient facilities, and hospitals that offer comprehensive telehealth solutions will be able to provide prospective patients with a clear differentiator from their competitors. Patients will want to use the group that offers more convenient care, more convenient follow-up appointments, and overall less expensive care through virtual consultations.

Telehealth solutions bring a new competitor *and* a new differentiator to the game. Hospitals and physician groups that fail to successfully implement telehealth solutions will see a loss in case volume to new telehealth providers as well as local groups that offer these innovative solutions. Hopefully, increasing the options for patients enables them to take more control of their health care. It gives them more choices for care, so they can choose the right provider at the right price for their specific needs.

Changing Regulations

Widely used telehealth changes the health care landscape dramatically. And regulations will need to adapt and catch up to adequately protect patients and medical practitioners. There are a few speculations currently about how telehealth might change medical regulations.

First, some people think that telehealth might pave the road for national regulations and licensing as opposed to state by state. Currently, each state regulates the medical practice. But having fifty different sets of rules, licensing fees, and definitions of what constitutes practicing medicine does not make as much sense in the era of telehealth. To patients, it merely seems like annoying red tape that hampers their ability to get medical care. For example, at the Mayo Clinic, doctors do follow up with patients virtually after in-person appointments. But people come to the Mayo Clinic from all over the country because of its reputation. In the current regulatory system, the doctors can only discuss the specific condition that was treated at the in-person visit. Any other new problem or concern cannot be discussed if the patient lives out-of-state (unless the doctor happens to be licensed in that state as well). Instead, the patient will need to come back to the Mayo Clinic in person or visit a local physician. While most states still want control over their medical regulations, licensing may be a good place to start. Some states currently have a program that allows a doctor in one state to quickly obtain a license in another state in this group. Hopefully more states will enact this type of solution, or perhaps a national license will be created.

Secondly, there may be more stringent definitions of "practicing medicine" in the eyes of the law. With the rise of the Internet, there are more and more companies that give advice and information that looks a lot like medical advice, but then they have fine print disclaimers stating that they are not US-licensed doctors. To protect consumers, a national regulation defining "practicing medicine" may need to be developed and implemented.

Lastly, another area that telehealth affects is payment models. As discussed in detail throughout the book, different telehealth solutions have different payment models. While our solution, as an independent provider, has a unique viewpoint on payment structure, telehealth solutions that, for example, are provided by hospitals need to fit a more traditional payment model. But insurers and Medicare and Medicaid are lagging in reimbursement laws for virtual consultations. As telehealth gets more popular, these reimbursement laws have to change. Luckily, it fits in well with the current trend towards fee-for-value care as opposed to fee-for-service. For example, a doctor will not be financially penalized for virtual follow-ups instead of in-person follow-ups, as long as the outcomes are better or the same.

Health Care of the Future

Telehealth will have far-reaching impacts on the current health care system that we can only begin to understand. While some are obviously good, such as lower costs for patients to access care, some will challenge hospitals and doctors to change their models to stay financially sound and relevant in the changing market. Laws and regulations will also have to change, and we can only hope that the laws change to enhance technological progress and increase access in health care while still protecting patients.

CHAPTER 15

Telepsychiatry - An Industry in Need

One of the most popular and fastest growing forms of telehealth is telepsychiatry—the use of telecommunications technology to provide mental and behavioral health services. Psychiatry and other mental health services are unique to other medical fields because they do not require touching or physically examining a patient. This makes these fields especially ideal for being delivered remotely. Furthermore, psychiatry is an industry in need, as demand has rapidly increased.

In the United States, the population that could benefit from mental health services has risen steadily over the past few decades. However, the number of psychiatrists has not grown at the same pace. This has resulted in a shortage of providers to meet the growing demand for services. The problem is especially acute in rural areas, where there may be as little as one doctor serving a large geographic area. In fact, a recent analysis by the US Health Resources and Services Administration projected that to meet the expected growth in demand by 2025, there would need to be an additional ten thousand providers in *each* of seven different mental health care professions. Besides the physician shortage, which is affecting most health care specialties, recent changes in coverage for mental health services has also affected demand. In 2008, the Mental Health Parity and Addiction Equity Act required all health care plans to establish the same deductibles, co-payments, and limits for mental health services as for other medical services. More recently, the Affordable Care Act gave many more people coverage, and all plans sold under the ACA must cover mental health and substance-abuse treatment.

There is also increasing recognition of the importance of behavioral and mental health, in both the consumer and medical fields. In the consumer space, wellness has become a key trend. Yoga and mindfulness have exploded in popularity. There are apps, trackers, and products all designed with self-care and reducing stress in mind. All of these consumer touchpoints have made more people conscious of their mental health. This has led to an abundance of online resources and mental health diagnostic tools that have increased the number of people looking for counseling or coaching. In the medical sphere, doctors, hospitals, health insurance companies, and employers are all starting to realize the importance of mental health. Research has shown that even mild to moderate mental health issues, if left untreated, can lead to additional health problems down the road.

But getting care, like in other specialties, is expensive and inconvenient for most patients. And since these are chronic conditions, patients are even more likely to postpone, often indefinitely, or skip treatments. According the National Alliance on Mental Illness, only 41 percent of adults with a mental illness received treatment in 2016. At the worst, these untreated patients could end up in a downward spiral, possibly even ending in an emergency room or in the criminal justice system. At the best, it results in more missed work, lower productivity, and worse overall health. To better serve many of these patients, telepsychiatry is a leading resource to provide cost-effective and convenient care.

How Telepsychiatry Works

Telepsychiatry is a natural extension of telehealth. After all, most therapy sessions are based on conversation and observation, both of which can be done via videoconference. That is why study after study has shown that telepsychiatry has equivalent outcomes to in-person sessions.

There are two main types of telepsychiatry. The first, and most basic, is a telemedicine solution provided by a patient's in-person provider or facility. These solutions allow patients to use both in-person and remote counseling sessions with the same provider, based on whatever is most convenient or appropriate at a given time. The second is a direct-to-consumer model, in which telehealth companies provide a platform for patients to speak with a remote provider. While the provider will be licensed in that patient's state, he or she is likely not available for additional in-person visits. With most stand-alone telehealth solutions, this is the model provided. It allows patients to speak immediately with a provider, so they can get care right when they are thinking about it and need it. While some solutions provide access to multiple specialties, mental health being just one, there are other companies that specialize in only telepsychiatry.

More and more companies are starting to provide telepsychiatry services because of how successful these programs are. Telepsychiatry is uniquely positioned for success because it can actually be better than in-person sessions. A key factor in the success of therapy is how open a patient is willing to be. And luckily, it has been found that many patients are *more* open with their counselor in a virtual session than an in-person session. While there is no way to pinpoint exactly why, patients may feel more comfortable in their own home. They may be less stressed about trying to fit the appointment in during a busy day. Or having a bit of distance between them and the provider may be what makes them more comfortable. Regardless, it seems to work better for some patients.

Additionally, some providers report benefits of seeing patients in their natural environment. These providers get to see patients in their home—even if unintentionally, providers often get a peripheral view of their living space or perhaps even a family member. It can provide great context for providers to help paint a better and perhaps more realistic picture of their patient's life.

While there are benefits to the actual therapy sessions themselves, the biggest benefit to telepsychiatry is improved access. As discussed, there is not enough supply to meet the current, and growing, demand for services. By using telepsychiatry, physicians are better able to meet the demands. And patients have more convenient access to care, regardless of their location or their access to reliable transportation. This makes them more likely to get care in the first place and then makes them less likely to miss appointments in the future.

In particular, this improved access to care benefits those groups in areas that have additional difficulties with access to care. This includes schools, colleges, jails, and mild to moderately ill patients.

Telepsychiatry in Schools and Colleges

One in five children ages thirteen to eighteen have or will have a serious mental illness. Fifty percent of all lifetime mental illnesses begin by age fourteen, and 75 percent begin by age twenty-four. But the average delay between onset of symptoms and intervention is eight to ten years. Fifty percent of students that are fourteen and older and have a mental illness will drop out of high school.[16]

These are sobering statistics. Most people know that the transition from childhood to adolescence and on to adulthood is challenging. But for many students, these challenges result in mental health problems that can last for the rest of their lives if left untreated. And unfortunately, this population is often underserved and faces unique challenges in seeking mental health care.

Many of these children and teens are not in control of their health care or finances. They may not know the difference between in-network and out-of-network providers. They probably do not have the money to seek treatment on their own. Parents may not support treatment, either emotionally or financially. Some have a "suck it up" attitude. Others will not drive children to and from sessions or agree to pay for them. Children and teens may not even share their struggles with their parents, due to fear or shame.

This age group is also not as emotionally mature or knowledgeable about mental health problems. While schools are teaching students how to recognize depression and suicidal thoughts, other problems that can be effectively treated with therapy, such as anxiety or OCD, are usually not discussed. Students are often not as aware of warning signs and symptoms. Over the course of their lives, many adults know people who have struggled with anxiety or depression. Many adults have more perspective and know that these feelings are normal and can be treated, but children and teenagers often feel very alone. They may avoid talking to parents or peers about it because they feel embarrassed.

Because of these unique challenges, schools and colleges are finding themselves as crucial touchpoints for students' mental health. Students already come to class almost every day, and teachers and school counselors may be more aware of symptoms and changes in behavior. Unfortunately, hiring a psychologist or psychiatrist is expensive and not in most schools' budgets. Most schools would not have the volume of cases needed to support a full-time employee, either. Some schools want to rely heavily on their counselor, but that is not truly a school counselor's role. Most school counselors are focused on career development and college applications and preparation. They also help mediate conflicts between peers and between students and teachers. They run clinics on bullying, sex education, and study skills. While one-on-one counseling for anxiety, depression, and ADHD are available, they are not usually the best contact for these services. Not only are those areas not their specialty, but these mental illnesses are best served by a counselor or therapist who is *outside* of the school. School counselors, especially in smaller schools, have prejudices and ingrained opinions about the patient, other students, and teachers that are almost impossible to suspend during sessions.

Instead, schools and colleges are starting to rely more heavily on telepsychiatry services. This enables them to have access to the proper professionals in any instance. School counselors can connect a student in need with a telepsychiatrist who can help them over a longer period and on the student's schedule. If the student has access to his or her own technology, the student can even have sessions outside of school hours. Otherwise, the school can provide a private room for the sessions. Students in particular can benefit from telepsychiatry because they are tech savvy and used to videoconferencing. They are unlikely to get flustered from troubleshooting and will feel comfortable talking to the screen. Their unique challenges, high need for services, and comfort with technology make them perfect candidates for telepsychiatry services.

Telepsychiatry in Prisons

Prisons are another group that poses a challenge for mental health care. The majority of inmates at prisons would benefit from mental health counseling. But there are difficulties in providing care. Either the doctors or counselors have to come to the prison or the inmates have to be transported to the provider.

Not all providers want to drive to the correctional facility. It takes time out of their day, and there is a danger, real or perceived, of interacting with patients. Typically, a guard will need to be present, which makes the patient unlikely to open up with the counselor. On the other side, most providers do not want inmates in their private facilities, due to worry for the safety and security of their facility and their other patients. With telepsychiatry, these problems are eliminated. The inmates can get the care they need without inconvenience or safety issues for the providers.

Many prisons have already implemented telepsychiatry solutions to great success. Ohio, Texas, Arizona, and Georgia are all success stories that teach us how telepsychiatry has been effective. Findings include that telepsychiatry helps inmates feel more satisfied with their health care, causing them to file fewer grievances. The reduction in paperwork and man hours for grievance procedures saved a significant amount of money. The availability of telepsychiatry also led more patients to seek these services, perhaps due to the perceived ease and the lack of having to see someone in person. Some inmates are more comfortable being removed from their provider.

While studies are still early, researchers hope to prove that telepsychiatry improves outcomes in prisons and reduces recidivism. In the meantime, the cost savings and improved inmates' perceptions are reason enough to expand and continue these programs.

Telepsychiatry for the Mildly to Moderately Ill

More and more doctors are starting to see the importance of mental health care for those with mild to moderate mental illnesses. These are the patients who are suffering from a mental illness but are able to maintain a decent level of normalcy in their lives. Sometimes these are chronic, low-level conditions that emerged in childhood or adolescence. Other times, they are brought on by traumatic events or difficult life changes. Some people will function at this level throughout their entire lives, never seeking care but never getting worse either. Others will spontaneously recover. Still others will spiral into severe mental illness. With the strong connection between severe mental illness and death, for example alcoholism with accidental death or depression with suicide, treating patients at the outset of symptoms may be a more effective way to treat the mentally ill population.

Telepsychiatry helps this group in particular because it reduces the barriers to care. Reduction in cost is part of the solution, but more important is the stigma and the convenience. Mental illnesses still carry a strong stigma. Many people are uncomfortable about admitting a problem or seeking help. Especially with mild mental illness, many people feel their problems are not bad enough to warrant a conversation with a therapist. But picking up the phone or videoconferencing a counselor from your own home can help reduce the fear of the stigma. A patient does not have to worry about anyone seeing him or her at a mental health facility. And there is something about a phone call that seems less serious than an in-person visit (even though its proven to be as effective!). It is also easier to fit into a person's schedule. People struggling with mental illnesses often struggle with motivation. And people are genuinely busy. Being able to eliminate travel time makes it easy for a patient to schedule a session and makes him or her less likely to postpone or skip treatments.

Furthermore, many mild to moderate mental illnesses do not require extensive psychotherapy. A few initial sessions may be enough to help the patient develop self-monitoring skills and behavioral adjustments. After that, the patient may only need periodic check-ins to assess any new developments and how treatment is going. But by having an easy way for patients to access mental health care, the hope is that more mental health problems will be addressed sooner, reducing problems later in life and improving quality of life sooner for these patients.

Therapy on Demand

Mental health is serious. While most people would not skip a doctor's appointment for a broken bone, people skip or avoid doctor's appointments for depression and anxiety all the time. But poor mental health is associated with countless negative outcomes. With telepsychiatry, especially on-demand telepsychiatry, patients can access the mental health care they need *now*. It helps all patients, but especially those who have extra difficulties receiving in-person care. It is a great opportunity for technology to transform psychiatry and to help more people lead happy, healthy lives.

CHAPTER 16

Other Emerging Specialties

Direct-to-consumer telehealth first developed as a solution to bring primary care to patients as an alternative to costly urgent cares and emergency rooms. But as the concept gains traction and technology improves, telehealth companies, physicians, and consumers have all realized the potential that telehealth has to bring convenient specialty care to a larger population. Doctors in these specialty fields have begun to embrace the technology and its ability to improve access and continuity of care within their practice. And telehealth providers have begun to add access to these specialties to their existing on-demand solutions. Telepsychiatry may be the easiest and most complete specialty that telehealth can replicate, but other specialties such as physical therapy, dentistry, and optometry have more use cases that can be served by telehealth than you may think.

Physical Therapy
If you or anyone you know has had an injury that required physical therapy treatment, you know firsthand how time consuming

and expensive it can be. It usually takes *at least* four weeks of treatment and can be up to sixteen weeks or more. And did I mention that you have homework of the exercises to complete at home? The exercises are, at best, boring and time consuming (think a sprain) and at worst, painful and frustrating (think about a knee replacement). Each visit, even with insurance, can cost between ten and seventy-five dollars. That adds up quickly over the course of many weeks. Progress is often slow. Patients get used to their current level of mobility, and life gets busy. So it's no surprise that most patients do not complete all of their physical therapy appointments. All of this makes physical therapy a prime opportunity for telehealth.

Like other telehealth specialties, remote physical therapy can take multiple forms, depending on the provider and the patient needs. For serious injuries and postoperative physical therapy, patients will likely need to see an in-patient physical therapist as well. Typically, the first meeting will be in person, as well as periodically throughout the healing process. But after that first meeting, instead of weekly or biweekly in-person appointments that are time consuming and likely to be skipped, the patient can have virtual appointments instead. Using a video-enabled telemedicine device, the physical therapist can watch the patient perform specific exercises and provide feedback. The physical therapist can ask questions about progress and pain levels, using this information to adjust or modify the exercises, if necessary. These visits help the physical therapist ensure that the patient is making progress and actually doing the homework exercises. Patients get to resolve questions about exercises more quickly and have more frequent and more convenient feedback. Overall, supplementing in-person physical therapy appointments with remote visits leads to higher patient engagement and reduced absenteeism, both of which help improve outcomes.

For less serious injuries, a completely virtual physical therapy program could be effective. This is where on-demand physical therapists are especially helpful. For example, neck and lower back pain from long hours at a desk is a common complaint with easy at-home exercises that a physical therapist could talk through with the patient without a hands-on assessment. If the patient has follow-up questions, the patient could reach a physical therapist right away instead of waiting for the next scheduled appointment. Many patients have questions about specific exercises the first time they have to do them on their own. Instead of perhaps doing an exercise incorrectly for an entire week, the question and form could be addressed quickly, making progress faster. Other examples of common injuries would be mild carpal tunnel, shin splints, or plantar fasciitis.

Another type of physical therapy telehealth that is rapidly gaining traction combines a video library of exercises with virtual consultations with a physical therapist. With these services, patients can meet with a physical therapist to discuss symptoms and get a diagnosis and an at-home exercise plan. Then, the patient can access the video library to get detailed videos on how to correctly perform the exercises. If the patient still has questions, he or she can speak with an on-demand physical therapist as well. Some in-person physical therapy offices are also utilizing video libraries of exercises, as they are an easy way to reduce patient questions and improve outcomes.

An even more sophisticated version of telehealth enabled physical therapy is through game-console systems that actually track a patient's movements, such as the Microsoft Kinect. These systems were originally developed for video game consoles, so that players could physically interact with a video game. But this same technology has been adapted to facilitate at-home rehab. The system can provide a gamified version of rehabilitative exercises, making compliance more likely. It can also track patient data to send to the rehabilitation team so that the team can assess and adjust programs when necessary. Not only does this solution enable patients to remain at home for their rehab, but it also significantly reduces costs and keeps patients engaged.

All of these services make physical therapy more affordable and more convenient, improving program adherence, which is especially difficult in physical therapy.

Dentistry

Of all specialties, dentistry may at first appear to be a stretch for virtual care. How much can really be done remotely? That is why telehealth in dentistry is widely used in conjunction with other medical visits, but it can also be used in remote appointments to treat minor dental concerns.

One of the most widely discussed innovations in teledentistry is programs that connect dental hygienists throughout a community to a central dentist. In California and Colorado, these virtual dentistry programs have been implemented to great success. In rural areas, there may not be a conveniently located dentist. And there are not enough dentists to effectively travel throughout the region, not to mention that it would be cost prohibitive. So in these programs, dental *hygienists* are deployed to community settings (churches, community centers, schools) to provide preventive dental-care services. Dental hygienists can provide routine cleanings as well as information and tools on proper dental care. But that is not all. The dental hygienists are connected with a central dentist via telecommunications technology. The dental hygienist can post radiographs, intraoral photographs, and chartings for the dentist to review. The dentist can evaluate and plan treatment, as well as direct the dental hygienist in any additional care that is within their scope. There are many interim restorations or care than can be done by a hygienist until the patient can schedule a visit with a dentist. This model closely replicates most traditional in-person regular dental visits. Typically, the dental hygienist performs the cleanings, photos, x-rays, and chartings. Only at the end of the visit does the dentist come in to review. This remote model allows the dentist to perform the review remotely, only bringing in patients that really need further care. It helps reduce costs and provide convenient care to remote and underserved populations.

Telehealth can also reduce the need for specialty visits by enabling dentists to consult with a specialist remotely. Orthodontics is a great example of this. There are actually a wide range of cases that dentists are capable of handling but may not be as comfortable with. Instead of an unnecessary referral to an orthodontist, the dentist could consult with an orthodontist remotely for some quick advice. With the orthodontist's recommendation and tips, the dentist could treat the patient immediately. Dentists could also consult with TMJ experts, oral surgeons, and prosthodontists, for example. By linking dentists with these specialists, dentists become more empowered to provide care. It also reduces the travel and time burden for patients by reducing the number of visits required to get the care they need.

There are also instances where remote consultations from home with a dentist can be useful as well. Minor dental problems, such as a toothache, canker sores, or rubber ligature displacement on braces are all examples of conditions that can be diagnosed and treated, as least temporarily, via a remote consultation.

Poor dental health is linked with many other negative health outcomes. But many individuals in rural or low-income areas do not have access to the dental care they need. Telehealth dentistry has been proven to improve access and outcomes for these underserved patient populations.

Optometry

Optometry, like dentistry, is usually provided by an independent physician in a local office. While if you live in a city, there may be multiple eye doctors within a five-mile radius, in rural and low-income areas there may not be an optometrist anywhere nearby. But most Americans need the help of an optometrist or ophthalmologist at some point in their lives, and telehealth enabled optometry is helping to make eye care more convenient and accessible for all patients. Here is how telehealth is already being used in this field.

The first use is for improving communication with a patient's existing optometrist. Like most specialties, there are many surgeries that require follow-up appointments as well as chronic conditions that require regular, frequent monitoring. Both of these use cases can be streamlined by using telehealth. For surgeries, a great example is LASIK. LASIK surgery corrects nearsightedness, farsightedness, and astigmatism to improve a patient's vision without the need for glasses or contacts. This surgery is very common and highly successful, but it does currently require follow-up visits with the optometrist. Using telehealth, these visits can be reduced. A patient can videoconference with the eye doctor to discuss any problems or concerns instead of visiting in person. LASIK already requires a person to take off work for at least a day for the surgery. By enabling a patient to conduct a follow-up visit from home, it reduces the need to leave work or family to travel to the optometrist.

Optometrists also see many patients for chronic condition management, such as age-related macular degeneration and ocular surface disorders. These visits can become a burden to both patients and optometrists due to the amount of time these repetitive visits take. The visits are usually very routine, but they are necessary for identifying changes or problems quickly. But there are now telehealth solutions that help reduce the number of in-person visits needed by providing remote care instead. These solutions use a combination of self-reported evaluations and tests along with videoconferences with the optometrist to track eye health and catch any problems early. Early detection is key in many conditions, which makes this solution very valuable.

Appointments are less likely to be skipped, and problems requiring medical intervention can be identified and treated sooner. Patients are more engaged and can stay on top of their eye health.

Optometrists can also be useful in an on-demand remote setting. There are many minor, low-risk conditions that can be easily handled at home with a videoconference to an optometrist. Dry eye and burst blood vessels are two such conditions. Both are common, and optometrists have seen an increase in dry eye concerns, in particular. Because of the amount of time most people spend looking at screens in today's world, an increasing number of the population is dealing with dry eye symptoms. But this condition is easily diagnoses and treated via a remote consultation, and so is not worth the time or money that an in-person visit would require. Telehealth can reduce the burden of dry eye for both optometrists and patients. There are even platforms that have developed self-evaluation tests that can provide doctors with data they can use along with a consultation to develop a diagnosis and treatment plan.

Technology will keep improving and developing, expanding the scope of eye care that is able to be provided remotely. One of the most recent exciting advances in telemedicine-enabled optometry is the development of portable, self-operated vision testing devices. These are handheld devices accompanied with a software program that guides the user on how to perform the vision exam. These devices allow an ordinary consumer to order the right prescription lenses without visiting an optometrist. While too expensive for individual ownership, these devices can be conveniently located in pharmacies, hospitals, workplaces, and schools. It is a low-cost, convenient alternative that can help improve the vision of Americans without access to an optometrist.

Access to Specialties Improves Access to Care

As more and more specialties become available via telehealth, patients' access to care will improve, hopefully leading to better health outcomes. By connecting patients to specialists, patients can easily and quickly get medical questions answered and resolved, becoming more informed, engaged patients. These services help all patients, but especially those who struggle to access care today because of the prohibitive costs and logistic difficulties in reaching some of these specialists. It helps level the playing field for these groups, which is why it is so important to choose a telehealth provider that offers access to these specialists at no additional cost. By providing a solution that addresses as many specialties as possible, patients and consumers can get the most benefit from telehealth.

CHAPTER 17

The Future of Telehealth

At this stage, there are few people who doubt that telehealth will be an integral part of our future health care system. Technology has become second nature in many aspects of business and personal life; there's no reason that health care will not follow the same path. All of the drivers for change are there—fee-for-value care models, increased consumerism, and cost containment—but exactly what role telehealth will play in the future system is still unclear.

Telecommunications technology progressed rapidly, and new ideas are developing every day, unlocking tons of potential for innovation. Health care is only just beginning to embrace the new technologies and all of its possibilities. But with so many options for growth, no one knows quite how telehealth will develop. While it's impossible to know for certain what the future of telehealth is—after all, new improvements, new regulations, and new service models will all influence the future—there are many predictions and perspectives that shed light on where the industry is headed.

Integration versus New Providers

The greatest potential of telehealth lies in its ability to reduce the number of in-person visits, thus reducing the time and cost needed for care. There are two main viewpoints on how this should be done.

The first viewpoint is that telehealth's growth will come mainly from improving access to a patient's *existing* health network. Currently, the only way for many patients to engage with their hospital or doctor is in person. The patient calls his or her primary care doctor and schedules an appointment, typically weeks after the call. The first visit often results in a second visit. Either it's a follow-up visit to see how treatment, or a new medication is going, or maybe the patient is referred to a specialist. This process is slow and fragmented. Appointments can take weeks to schedule and are often inconvenient to the patient. Because of the time and cost involved, many patients simply skip follow-up appointments. The no-show rate ranges from 5 to 50 percent. It is a massive cost to the industry and leads to worse health outcomes. While telehealth cannot replace all follow-up appointments, it could drastically reduce the number of in-person follow-up appointments needed. For chronic condition management or when starting a new prescription, the patient could have a virtual follow-up quickly after the initial in-person visit. Questions, concerns about side effects, or reminders about treatment could be addressed quickly, instead of weeks later or not at all if the patient does not show up. Or when the examining physician thinks a specialist opinion is necessary, the specialist could be video conferenced in to the current appointment. Patients could avoid duplicate visits and could receive care quickly, instead of delaying a diagnosis for weeks until the specialist appointment. Increased use of telehealth could save individuals and the system valuable time and money, all while improving the continuity of care.

There are some doctors and hospitals that are already providing these services in limited capacity. In the future, connecting virtually with existing patients could be the norm. But hospitals are not technology experts. To deliver a seamless and friendly patient experience, they will need to engage with other companies. That is where telehealth providers come in. They will have the technical expertise to develop sophisticated platforms that meet patient and provider needs. In this scenario, many of these telehealth companies will be primarily behind-the-scenes technology providers instead of consumer-facing companies. Just as specific technology companies evolved to handle electronic health record requirements, telehealth technology companies and medical facilities will partner to provide telehealth services to their patient population. The telehealth provider will become an enabler for greater connectivity and information sharing in existing patient-physician relationships.

On the opposite side, some experts believe that telehealth providers will develop their own direct-to-consumer health care brand. Growth would come by redirecting nonemergency care to a virtual provider instead of an in-person doctor. In this view, telehealth companies are a stand-alone solution for consumers, not simply an add-on provided by an insurance company or hospital. Instead of using a virtual portal for a patient to connect with his or her existing doctor, telehealth providers would have their own network of doctors and their own brand to stand behind. These telehealth companies would be their own unique site of care, not just a third-party technology provider. Theoretically, someday a telehealth company could be as well-known as the Mayo Clinic.

While it may seem that these two visions of telehealth are conflicting, in reality they can both exist at the same time. They are complementary solutions that improve care, simply in different ways. Therefore, it is likely that different companies will evolve to serve both needs. Some companies may even evolve to provide both. Take, for example, Spectrum (formerly known as Time Warner Cable). Spectrum has a business side and a consumer side. Businesses need Internet and voice capabilities, as do individual home owners. People don't think about it, but when you leave a voice mail for a company, you're using their voice mail provider. Similarly, it is possible that telehealth companies will partner with hospitals as well as have a consumer-facing solution. Either way, it is clear that telehealth will improve access to care by reducing the number of in-person visits needed, whether that's a diagnosis for pinkeye or a follow-up appointment after starting a new medication.

New Services

Telehealth already has the capability to provide many services. There are primary care doctors who can diagnose and treat many common ailments, nutritionists and dietitians to provide weight loss and eating disorder counseling, pediatricians, psychologists, and more. But some telehealth companies are looking at how new services could expand the potential market for telehealth.

With telehealth's existing capabilities, there are a certain percentage of in-person visits that could be switched to a virtual visit. The previous growth models essentially want to increase their share of these visits. By adding new services, telehealth companies can increase the total percentage of in-person visits that telehealth could address.

One area that is already being explored is at-home lab testing. There are many common illnesses that can only be 100 percent accurately diagnosed with a lab test, such as strep throat and UTIs. But at-home diagnostic kits are being developed that would allow for fast and accurate results, all from a patient's home. Kits could be sold at local drugstores, or perhaps they could be delivered by services such as Amazon Prime Now, which can deliver in as little as one hour in certain areas.

As new technologies develop, so do the possibilities of health care from home. Could a smartphone camera detect eye problems? There is already an app that is working to diagnose concussions using just the smartphone camera. Could a breathalyzer detect particles in your breath that identify certain illnesses? The only limit for the future is your imagination. And each new technology enhances telehealth's potential.

Remote Data Collection

Another possibility for telehealth growth is improved use of remote data collection. We discussed remote patient monitoring and its current uses earlier in the book, but this is a field that has a lot of room to develop. Consumers have already embraced a multitude of health apps, tracking everything from steps to sleep. But the information collected is not necessarily shared with any medical professionals. The companies that develop these apps and devices have a lot of potential for going from a consumer tool to true telehealth providers.

Sleep disorders are a great example. Many patients complain that they feel sleep studies are inaccurate. After all, it is hard to have a normal night's sleep in an unfamiliar environment, hooked up to a bunch of different machines. But there are mattresses, wristbands, and other new trackers that are collecting data on how people sleep. The data is collected over time instead of just one night. Trends and averages can be developed, which are better indicators of frequency and severity of problems. This information could be used by sleep specialists to more accurately diagnose and treat a sleep disorder, without ever having to see a patient in person.

Many companies are already capitalizing on this market of consumer health tracking, but actual physician interaction and medical diagnosis is a missing component. Using the sleep disorder example, a mattress may be able to detect if you are sleeping more soundly on a firmer or softer mattress, but it will not connect you with a physician or provide a medical diagnosis. If someone chooses to go see a doctor, the doctor may or may not take any at-home data collection into account. Most likely, he or she will not. A patient's at-home treatments and diagnostics are usually happening independently of their interaction with a physician, even if it is for the same issue. By integrating these two distinct services, patients could be better engaged in their own health and have better health outcomes.

To really realize this vision, at least two things need to happen. First, the technologies need to improve and become more reliable. There will need to be rigorous testing to prove the concepts, especially if insurance is to reimburse any of the treatments or diagnostic tools. Second, physicians will need to be trained on the technologies and how to incorporate them into their practice. They need to be comfortable reading the outputs and understanding how they connect to a diagnosis and treatment plan. Clearly these are big hurdles to overcome, but the possibilities are exciting nonetheless. If the technology developers in this space choose to try to partner with the medical profession, this could be a huge area for growth in telehealth.

The Possibilities of Big Data

An inevitable piece of increased use of telehealth is increased data collection. Frequency of visits, health outcomes, and population health statistics will all be better captured using telecommunications technology. So the natural next step in telehealth is for telehealth providers to begin analyzing and synthesizing the data they are collecting.

The data being collected has a lot of potential for enhancing care. Sophisticated analytics could be able to identify especially at-risk patients earlier on. The data could be used to develop more personalized treatment plans. It could predict acute medical events, such as heart failure. It could forecast disease outbreak. It could even do more mundane things, such as speed up insurance approvals and payment turnarounds. All of these could transform the medical industry, reducing costs and improving the quality of care.

While many consumers dislike the idea of their health data being collected, it is easy for companies to deidentify the data so that it can be analyzed without affecting patient privacy concerns. Big data has revolutionized many industries and allowed for better decision making. Health care could certainly be next. Big data allows for data-driven insights and trend analysis so that the medical community can be better informed and can deliver better care. If telehealth technology providers can capitalize on the data they are collecting, they could evolve into true value drivers for the entire health care system.

The question is how this piece of the industry will develop. Will telehealth companies partner with big data companies to analyze their data? Or will telehealth companies develop their own sophisticated data and analytics teams within? Either way, big data collected by telehealth could lead to new insights and advances in health care.

Conclusion

There are a lot of roads telehealth could take in the future. As more and more people become familiar with technology and comfortable using it in their everyday lives, use of telehealth will spread further and further. Different experts and different companies have differing and sometimes competing visions for the future of telehealth. While they may not all develop as they think, it is exciting to see and hear about all of the potential telehealth technologies have for the future of health care.

It does seem that health care is often the last industry to embrace innovations, but that is only natural given that health is so important and personal. More companies are starting to push the envelope on how technology can improve access and communication in health care. And as a new generation of physicians develops that grew up with technology and a connected world, more and more medical facilities will embrace the innovations.

ABOUT THE AUTHOR

Larry Jones is chief executive officer and a member of the board of directors of TelaCare Health Solutions. Since starting the company in 2009, he has led TelaCare to its position today as one of the fastest growing telehealth companies, achieving significant growth in revenue, membership and telehealth utilization. Under his leadership the company has established a proven track record of successfully shaping the market and driving healthcare transformation by executing on the strategic vision and delivering award-winning innovation. Nationally recognized as a thought leader in the virtual delivery of healthcare, Larry Jones is fueled by a passion for improving healthcare outcomes and providing universal access to care.

In this position, Larry Jones has had the opportunity to use his background in computer science to transform how people access health care. He holds several trademarks and patents for different leading technologies used by many companies today. His experience has made him a highly sought after professional speaker in the technology arena. He has become one of the foremost leading technology experts and healthcare technology strategists.

During his 20-year career, he has pioneered the development of innovative technology services which evolved into mainstream offerings that simultaneously delivered meaningful value to customers and bottom-line business results. One of these technologies led to his creating MD Alert Project, Inc, a charity that helps connect people with chronic conditions with an emergency medical ID system called ViewMyID.

In addition to his role at TelaCare, Larry Jones is also CEO of several companies held under his holdings company. He is an expert in change management and technology adoption, with more than a dozen years of supporting diverse client organizations through transformational changes. He helps businesses develop enterprise scale and implement custom application platforms with proven scalability, performance, and reliability. His significant experience architecting and managing high performance projects and large relational database systems enables companies to improve performance.

Mr. Jones splits his time between central Indiana and Ohio. He has three kids and a loving wife. His drive and thirst for knowledge has led him to be a certified Krav Maga Instructor, Scuba Diving Instructor and DAN Instructor. He also enjoys mountain climbing and golf. He loves connecting with new people – if you want to talk technology, business, or hobbies, reach out to him on LinkedIn.

REFERENCES

1. Willis Towers Watson. *High-performance insights – best practices in health care.* 2017. https://www.willistowerswatson.com/-/media/WTW/PDF/Insights/2016/12/full-report-2016-21st-annual-willis-towers-watson-best-practices-in-healthcare-employer-survey.pdf

2. The Henry J. Kaiser Family Foundation and Health Research and Educational Trust. *Employer Health Benefits 2016 Annual Survey.* 2016. http://files.kff.org/attachment/Report-Employer-HealthBenefits-2016-Annual-Survey

3. IHS Markit. *The Complexities of Physician Supply and Demand 2017 Update: Projections from 2015 to 2030.* 2017. https://aamc-black.global.ssl.fastly.net/production/media/filer_public/a5/c3/a5c3d565-14ec-48fb-974b-99fafaeecb00/aamc_projections_update_2017.pdf

4. Peckham, Carol. *Medscape Physician Compensation Report 2016.* April 1, 2016. https://www.medscape.com/features/slideshow/compensation/2016/public/overview

5. Consumer Reports National Research Center. *Surprise Medical Bills Survey: 2015 Nationally-Representative Online Survey.* May 5, 2015. http://consumersunion.org/wp-content/uploads/2015/05/CY-2015-SURPRISE-MEDICAL-BILLS-SURVEY-REPORT-PUBLIC.pdf

6. World Health Organization. *Telemedicine: Opportunities and developments in Member States: Report on the second global survey on eHealth: Global Observatory for eHealth series – Volume 2.* 2010. www.who.int/goe/publications/goe_telemedicine_2010.pdf

7. "Telehealth". http://www.who.int/sustainable-development/healthsector/strategies/telehealth/en/

8. "About Telemedicine". http://www.americantelemed.org/about/telehealthfaqs-

9. CA Business and Professions Code, § 2290.5

10. "About Telemedicine". http://www.americantelemed.org/about/telehealthfaqs-

11. Aflac. *Aflac Workforces Report 2016: Employee Overview.* 2016. https://www.aflac.com/docs/awr/pdf/2016-overview/2016.awr_employee_findings_ebook.pc.pdf

12. Murphy, Kevin. *Is Telehealth becoming the new norm in patient care?.* June 11, 2015. www.poweredbyc2.com/2015/06/11/is-telehealthbecoming-the-new-norm-in-patient-care/

13. Willis Towers Watson. *High-performance insights – best practices in health care.* 2017. https://www.willistowerswatson.com/-/media/WTW/PDF/Insights/2016/12/full-report-

2016-21st-annual-willis-towers-watson-best-practices-in-healthcare-employer-survey.pdf

14. Wells Fargo Insurance Employee Benefits National Practice. *2016 Strategy, Actions, and Behaviors Study: Employee benefits trends in the workplace and marketplace.* December 2016. https://wfis.usi.com/insights/research/2016-Strategies-Actions-and-Behaviors-Study/Documents/2016-SABS-Employee-Benefits-Trends.pdf

15. Guttman, Dave. *29 Statistics You Need to Know About Healthcare & Telemedicine.* August 11 2017. https://www.fshealth.com/blog/29-statistics-about-telemedicine-healthcare

16. National Alliance on Mental Illness. *Mental Health By The Numbers.* https://www.nami.org/Learn-More/Mental-HealthBy-the-Numbers

Made in the USA
Middletown, DE
08 May 2018